A Phenomenological Interpretation of Schizophrenia

Pierluigi Parisi

A Phenomenological Interpretation of Schizophrenia

Subjectivation, Framework and Perspective

Springer

Pierluigi Parisi
Baden-Baden, Germany

ISBN 978-3-031-67859-2 ISBN 978-3-031-67860-8 (eBook)
https://doi.org/10.1007/978-3-031-67860-8

This Springer imprint is published by the registered company Springer Nature Switzerland AG
The registered company address is: Gewerbestrasse 11, 6330 Cham, Switzerland

Foreword

In this volume, the author develops a novel, philosophically grounded theory of schizophrenia and its underlying disorder, which he considers a fundamental loss of the order of human experience characterized by the key concepts of "perspectivity," "frame," and "subjectivity." Together, these terms denote the fundamental character of conscious experience, namely being intentionally directed toward the world from a center of awareness. This orientation of subjectivity concerns embodiment, spatiality, temporality, and intersubjectivity. Accordingly, the concepts of perspective and frame can be understood in multiple senses: literally, as in the case of creative art ("pictorial perspective," "pictorial frame") or metaphorically as, for instance, in the talk of "meaning frame," "situational frame," "interpretive frame," "interlocutor's perspective," and "temporal perspective."

The originality and creativity of the conception consists of using the three terms as "passepartouts," so to speak, which allow us to consider the most diverse, often disparate phenomena and symptoms of schizophrenia from an integrating point of view. These include loss of metaphorical language use (the so-called concretism), disorders of expressive comprehension, impairment of perspectival perception, or fragmentation of the experience of objects in space and time. The method used is phenomenological and interpretive, drawing on a wealth of empirical research findings and re-seeing and re-organizing them in the conception of frame and perspective. The various phenomena are finally synthesized into a comprehensive picture of schizophrenia as a disorder of the intentional frame of subjectivity, and as such linked to intersubjectivity: "Because schizophrenia destroys the ability to act within shared frames and perspectives, schizophrenia is a disorder of being-with."

With this fundamental analysis, the author makes an extremely valuable contribution to the understanding of a psychiatric disease that has remained puzzling and disturbing to this day. Precisely for this reason, however, the study and explanation of schizophrenia cannot be limited to neurobiological partial causes. Rather, integrative, superordinate conceptions are indispensable for a comprehensive understanding and for a holistic treatment of patients. In particular, these conceptions can provide an important conceptual basis for psychotherapeutic, art-based, and body-related treatment methods.

The theory of schizophrenia as an impairment of the basal bodily self-experience, which is currently significant in the phenomenological field, receives a significant addition and expansion with Pierluigi Parisi's conception. It will benefit all who are theoretically and practically concerned with the understanding and treatment of people with schizophrenia. Thus, it is to be hoped that this book will attract a wide and interested readership.

Department of General Psychiatry
Heidelberg University Hospital
Heidelberg, Germany

Thomas Fuchs

Karl Jaspers Professor for Philosophical Foundations of Psychiatry
Heidelberg, Germany

Preface

Basic Idea and Framework of the Book

In recent years I have become interested in the crisis affecting all aspects of social and cultural life, particularly the moral, social, economic, legal, medicinal, and artistic aspects. In pursuing my intuitions considering the possibility of establishing a diagnosis for the Western postmodern condition, I have applied methods garnered from a range of fields encompassing human behavior, language, art, and psychology, and have synthesized what I consider to be a new hypothetical worldview in which research regarding schizophrenia across these fields can give us some new insights. For instance, the German terms *Staat* (state), *Institution* (institution), *Statut* (statute), *Stadt* (city), *Stein* (stone), *Statue* (statue), *Stehen* (standing), *Verstehen* (understanding), or in Italian the terms *costituzione* (constitution), *stabile architettonico* (building), *stabilire* (to establish), *statuire* (to establish by decree or law) are just a few examples of terms that make it possible to analyse the current crisis of today's state, sculpting, urban planning, law, pedagogy, as well as of contemporary architecture, music, literature, theater, economy, and other fields in comparison with the past. Thus, through a linguistic analysis we can frame the general diagnosis of postmodernism. We can perceive that the current crisis of the Occident can be reduced to a crisis of the verbal root *sthā*, which has declined in all its possible manifestations. At this point I have shown how the protean and multifaceted crisis we face can be synthetically attributed to a crisis of stability, which then manifests itself in the fields of knowledge and human action. The term *stability* comes from the verbal root *sthā*. What has developed into a crisis in postmodern culture generally refers to the intrinsic meanings of the root *sthā*: The paradigms of verticality, hierarchy, and stable implementation. Whilst the original meaning of the root *sthā* ontologically is an existential one rooted in the discarding of classical metaphysics, the diagnosis of *sthā* as an ontological crisis follows logically from our interpretation. To make distinctions means to create and set boundaries and borders. To distinguish between what is morally right and what is morally wrong is to draw a defining line between right and wrong, appropriate and inappropriate. In so doing, our act of clarification involves boundary setting. At the geopolitical level also nation states are defined by borders within which law is exercised. What is important, is that the root *sthā* is the ontological means of difference. From a cognitive and gnoseological perspective any form of knowledge also presupposes difference.

Of the Absolute, as *ab-solutus* (i.e., separate from everything), one can indeed have no knowledge.

Our next consideration is: How can one show the crisis of, say, root and difference in the phenomenology of contemporary culture?

Having introduced the root *sthā* as a form of synthetic and analytical description of human culture and established *sthā* as a tool to reflect the importance of distinction and boundaries, we can now introduce the cultural tool of the frame that embodies these distinctions and boundaries. The frame is the linguists' tool that, when applied to art and human behavior, unifies and privileges location, differences and boundaries in one linguistic and artistic paradigm. It offers immense explanatory power in Western languages, not only because it materially distinguishes art from everything that is not art, but also because it metaphorically references areas of humanity to all areas and forms of human experience, both action and interaction. In the German language, the terms *Rahmenbedingungen* (framework conditions), *Rahmenprogramm* (framework program), *Rahmengesetz* (framework law), *Rahmenerzählung* (frame narrative) are examples of that. The word *Krankheitsbild* (clinical picture) is also an image where the signs and symptoms of a particular illness or condition are within the frame and everything that is not part of the frame remains outside the frame. It is important to emphasize that the frame is the symbolic and ontological-hermeneutic means of establishing difference, i.e., of any valid and stable human knowledge and experience.

From a historical and material point of view, the notion of a framed painting emerged in the late 16th century with the emergence and flourishing of the Italian Renaissance. The framed painting is a window on the world through which the artist's eye opens to the objective representation of nature. It is no coincidence that the modern perspective and the notion of a framed painting emerged in the Italian Renaissance. The art of the Renaissance discards the previous ways of painting in favor of a new representation of nature and landscape. The earlier two-dimensional representations of the Medieval period are replaced by three-dimensional representation of landscapes. The Italian Renaissance brings to life not only the perspective and the physically framed image but also introduces an awareness of humanity located at the center of this world of sense experience and knowledge. At this moment, for the Renaissance human being, standing as they are on the threshold of Modernity, the concepts of subjectivity, perspective and frame represent a novel yet indissoluble and clear unity of subject and object.

Over the last three years I have been philosophically developing a phenomenological diagnosis of the crisis of subjectivity in Western postmodernity: The loss of stability of subjectivity corresponds to a crisis of both perspective and frame. What is fundamental to consider now is that subjectivity in all its individual, political, institutional, legal and other forms is closely linked to perspective and frame. These too are to be understood in their visual and material as well as their metaphorical sense.

Thus, we return to our psychopathological analysis, albeit on a historical, philosophical, anthropological, artistic, architectural, legal, economic and social, level. Subjectivity manifests itself in both perspective and frame, and the crisis, the absence, the impairment of subjectivity presents itself as a loss of perspective and frame. What can be said about the psychopathology of schizophrenia in relation to perspective and frame, considering the fact that schizophrenia is the psychiatric disorder in which subjectivity is most impaired?

The analytical process I have pursued in recent years became inductive once I was able to intuitively understand the principles of subjectivity, perspective and frame. Now I am able to follow a new deductive form of analysis. Given the historical, philosophical and cultural universality of this principle in the broadest sense, is it possible to reject it in the psychopathological field and specifically with respect to schizophrenia?

In view of this general working hypothesis, I expect that by analyzing art, behavior, spoken language, body language, and perception of space and time in schizophrenia, I will encounter problems associated with the concepts of perspective and frame, both in a concrete and metaphorical sense.

If this attempt should succeed, then we will have established a new relationship between philosophy and psychiatry.

Baden-Baden, Germany Pierluigi Parisi

The original version of this book has been revised. About the Author and a Foreword by Thomas Fuchs have been included in the book. Corrections have been made on pages iv, v and ix.

Acknowledgements

I would like to extend my sincere thanks to Alexandra Bakowski and Jan Wilkinson for the realizing of the English version of this book.

Special gratitude to Prof. Dr. Dr. Thomas Fuchs for the role he and his institute play in international research in psychopathology and phenomenological philosophy.

Contents

About the Author

Pierluigi Parisi

His research focuses on interpreting contemporary epochs, drawing inspiration from an interdisciplinary and multi-perspective approach that incorporates insights from ancient Greek and Italian Renaissance thought. Since 2016, he has been working on a general philosophical theory and phenomenological description of contemporary issues. Pierluigi Parisi, a polyglot, gave his first conference at the age of 16 and his first university lecture at the age of 21. Over the past 20 years, he has lectured on many different topics of culture and the human condition. His publications have appeared in scientific books and articles in Italian, English, and German. His thinking has been enriched by countless encounters with intellectuals and Nobel Prize winners from different disciplines.

Pierluigi Parisi attended the Conservatory of Music in Lecce, where he earned a Diploma in Teoria and Solfeggio. He also holds degrees in Medicine and Surgery from the Università Cattolica del Sacro Cuore in Rome, Philosophy from both Università del Salento in Lecce and Università di Trento, Mariology from the Pontificia Facoltà Teologica Marianum in Rome, History of Art and History of Architecture, as well as Ethno-Anthropology, from the Università La Sapienza in Rome, and Legal Sciences at the Università degli Studi di Bari in Taranto. He also holds two doctorates, one in Medicine from the Universität Heidelberg and another in Philosophy from the Pontificia Universitas Gregoriana in Rome.

1 Introduction

1.1 Topic and Research Question

The main topic of this book is a psychiatric disorder that has fascinated physicians throughout history. Even though schizophrenia is both medically and life-worldly prototypical of what humanity has always referred to as "madness," the nosological definition of this psychiatric pathology only emerged as late as the nineteenth century with Kraepelin and Bleuler.

Over the last few decades, there has been an enormous growth in scientific studies looking at very different aspects of this condition. Using ever more subtle research methods, linguists have attempted to analyze the discourse of persons with schizophrenia in order to analyze how persons with schizophrenia communicate: Their use of syntax, the coherence of conversations, and their ability to focus on a particular topic during a conversation or to integrate a text into a social context represent just some aspects of the themes that psychiatrists and linguists have been jointly exploring.

Modern technologies for studying human and animal behavior have also been used in this psychopathological field. Some researchers have devoted many of their studies to examine the way schizophrenia patients behave, use gestures, move, or communicate with their body language and signals. Likewise, studying the facial expressions, proxemics, and body language of individuals with schizophrenia has yielded useful data regarding their relationships and social behavior.

In this way, the classical clinical observations on schizophrenia have been expanded and reinterpreted in recent decades with much new experimental data.

The increasing amount of information from the analysis of drawings and paintings created by individuals with schizophrenia, such as those found in the Heidelberg Prinzhorn Collection Museum, has also played an important role in the interpretation. Although some individuals with schizophrenia are not recognized in the world of art as artists in the true sense of the word, others have become famous thanks to the publication of their artwork. In this book, all drawings and paintings by patients

P. Parisi, *A Phenomenological Interpretation of Schizophrenia*,
https://doi.org/10.1007/978-3-031-67860-8_1

with schizophrenia will be referred to as "works of art," even if this expands the conventional artist's concept of art.

Nevertheless, *schizophrenia* remains puzzling for psychopathologists, since it is an umbrella term that encompasses very different forms of the same pathology. Different patients offer different clinical pictures. Psychopathologists are confronted with a huge and diverse amount of data and scientific studies on schizophrenia and can sometimes be at a loss in *how to make sense out of the huge amount of data that has become available.* Is it possible to find a convincing link between the different symptomatologic islands of the clinical archipelago of schizophrenia? Is it possible to create a consistent model that would serve as a compass and allow a consistent interpretation of the data with such a diversity of symptoms manifest in the clinical presentation? To continue the compass metaphor: To which polestar should the psychopathologists' gaze be directed in order to better orient themselves in the many clinical and symptomatic constellations? These questions have motivated the investigation that will be presented in this book.

Here, the relevance of philosophical reflection for medical practice and especially for the psychopathology of schizophrenia becomes apparent. The polestar we are looking for cannot be sought by looking at the horizon or the waves of the sea, but by looking into the clear sky of theory. Only a theoretical orientation can help shed light on a landscape that is forever different and changing. The polarstar followed in this investigation can be outlined by the basic concepts of *subjectivity*, *frame*, and *perspective*.

These three terms are the facets that form a hermeneutic prism through which it will be possible to observe and evaluate the various clinical presentations of schizophrenia. Given that subjectivity is profoundly disturbed and impaired in schizophrenia patients, we can hypothesize that the impairment of subjectivity can be interpreted as an impairment of frame and perspective. What does this mean? The terms *frame* and *perspective* are of enormous interpretive importance because of their semantic potential. *Frame* and *perspective* can be understood in multiple senses, as in the case of figurative art, or in metaphorical senses, as exemplified in the German terms like *Bedeutungsrahmen* (frame of meaning), *Situationsrahmen* (situational frame), *sozialer Rahmen* (social frame), *Perspektive des Gesprächsparters* (perspective of the interlocutor), or *zeitliche Perspektive* (temporal perspective).

1.2 Design of the Study

The study presented here is divided into five chapters, each covering the areas of research and offering a clinical presentation showing how the field has progressively developed. Using this structure, we will explore the signs and symptoms of schizophrenia as they can be seen in the patients' linguistic, artistic, and gestural forms of expression. Each chapter presents two levels of analysis using two foci.

The first chapter gives an overview of the topic followed by a detailed analysis which allows for a direct comparison with experimental evidence and observations from clinical practice and research. The second chapter is devoted to the analysis of speech and speech disorders in individuals with schizophrenia. Since the way of speaking reflects the speaker's way of thinking, analyzing the linguistic structures and expression of patients with schizophrenia can illuminate aspects of their perception and representation of the world that would otherwise remain hidden and unnoticed. Schizophrenia patients often have their own way of speaking in their manner of treating the subject of speech and their interactions with one or more people. In this context, the concepts of *perspective* and *situational frame* will prove useful in dealing with the peculiarities of discourse on the nature of schizophrenia. The frequently observed inability to comprehend metaphors indicates the difficulty in managing the semantic and cognitive frame within which a metaphorical expression should be interpreted. The inability to comprehend irony suggests that the patient has problems recognizing the situational frame of the discourse or the personal perspective of the speaker. The notion of the frame assists us in analyzing the discourse on schizophrenia in terms of overall cohesion and coherence. It is the frame of meaning that constitutes a meaningful and organic discourse because this discourse is, in a sense, organized as a uniform composition.

The third chapter introduces *micro-sociology,* the branch of sociology which starting with Goffman (1959) has been supporting the analysis of human behavior in everyday situations that involve few social actors. How do patients with schizophrenia interact in the social context? How do they present themselves to others through their emotions, their gaze, their proxemics, their facial expressions, and their body language? What do they understand about other people's emotions, their facial expressions, and their gestures? The chapter will look at experiments such as recording eye movements or interpreting body postures. Body language can thereby be analyzed as a language that has its own rules and codes of behavior inscribed in cultural and anthropological frames. Apart from the verbal language, patients with schizophrenia also present deficits in the non-verbal language, for instance an inability to master the entire range of gestures, facial expressions, and emotions. Understanding or expressing an emotion means being able to see a face holistically, that is, to say in its entirety and in its salient features. All of these aspects are usually impaired in schizophrenia.

The fourth chapter offers an analysis of the *drawings and paintings* of patients with schizophrenia who are occasionally acknowledged as gifted artists. Like linguistic expression, patients' gaze and manner of looking, their facial expressions, gestures, proxemics, as well as their artistic expression present us with a fertile field of study for understanding the perception and representation of the world of individuals with schizophrenia. The chapter analyzes artistic forms as symptomatic expressions of the patients' difficulties in dealing with figurative perspective, naturalistic representation, as well as the framing of the general and unified order of a composition.

The fifth chapter is dedicated to the pathological *perception of spatiality.* The world of individuals with schizophrenia may appear disrupted because the spatial relationship between objects is often experienced in a fragmented way. Phenomena such as microscopy and macroscopy, where objects are falsely visually perceived as very small or very large, can result from both the loss of the overall view (i.e., a breakdown of the frame) and the loss of an integrated spatial perspective. Seeing in unity and perspective means that estimating the size of objects depends on both the experience with the physical dimensions of the object and the estimation of the distance. Subject and object are not only closely related in visual perception; rather, when subjectivity is disturbed, then the entire perception of the real world is disturbed. For example, some experimental studies have shown that individuals with schizophrenia are often unable to perceive the surrounding space, a landscape, or a picture in its entirety. The focus on details impairs the holistic perception of space. Here, the concept of frame is also of great importance. The ability to perceive the real world as three-dimensional sometimes seems to be impaired in schizophrenia. This is revealed by experiments conducted using tests with optical illusions or video games.

The sixth chapter deals with the *experience of the temporal dimension.* This topic is addressed last because it has turned out to be the most complex one and because it results in a synthesis of the preceding chapters. Time is the most fundamental dimension of consciousness. Everything that is perceived or acted upon happens within the scope of time. To analyze the impairment of temporal perspective is to shed light on the impairment of the *ego* in individuals with schizophrenia. Although time has been a subject of debate since the beginning of the history of Western philosophy, this analysis will draw mainly on contemporary philosophers and will deal specifically with the clinical-phenomenological observations made by the psychiatrists of the twentieth century. Observing the dissolution of temporal structure will enable us to understand the destruction of *the self* and schizophrenic subjectivity.

1.3 Methods

The method used in this research is phenomenological, descriptive, and interpretive. Analyzing schizophrenic clinical phenomena means first putting aside theoretical ideas one has on the subject. In this way, it becomes possible to attempt to reorganize all knowledge about schizophrenia within the new subjective-perspectival frame theory that is presented and proposed here.

Thanks to this phenomenological method, it is possible to develop an innovative interpretation of the diverse schizophrenic symptomatology. This method is also optimal because it is suitable for the analysis of seemingly very heterogeneous aspects such as verbal language, nonverbal language, graphic representations, and perceptions of space and time.

The German art historian and scientist Aby Warburg has created with his *Pictorial Atlas Mnemosyne* (Warburg, 1929) a method that leads to a concept based on juxtaposed examples. Each picture in Warburg's *work* is an example of his concept. Between the concept and the concrete examples, there is both a break and an inherent connection. This outlined interplay of examples and concept corresponds to the abductive method in the sciences (Eco, 1999, p. 306). An abduction is a hypothetical conclusion arrived at from a study of the individual examples which yield a general theory that fits best with the available data and evidence. In this analysis, studies from different scientific fields are presented that examine the impairments in patients with schizophrenia. By looking at the examples of linguistic, social, and artistic expression, a holistic picture of schizophrenia develops as an emergent phenomenon.

In this book, studies, reflections, observations, and results are presented which gain their theoretical strength in a global and integrated interpretation. The triad of *subjectivity*, *perspective*, and *frame* transcends and is immanent in each example. All examples given here from the cases examined can fairly be described as representing an impairment of subjectivity, perspective, and frame.

1.4 Materials

This theoretical work is based on the analysis and elaboration of the results of existing experimental and clinical studies, including scientific articles, publications, books, papers, pictures, and drawings. The large number of studies referred to in this book is evidenced by extensive bibliographical references in the chapters and by the list of literature at the end. With the help of this corpus, the state of knowledge about schizophrenia with its various forms and many deficiencies was systematically examined. The sources are relatively heterogeneous, as they often come from different historical periods and from relatively autonomous disciplinary fields. The innovation of this work lies in the presenting of a unified picture of schizophrenia drawn from the evidence of these heterogeneous elements. For this purpose, the triad of *subjectivity*, *perspective*, and *frame* is used as a structuring dispositive principle.

Analysis of Language Behavior 2

2.1 Introduction

This chapter analyzes some basic aspects of language used by individuals with schizophrenia and shows that the various impairments that become apparent can be summarized and interpreted by the terms *perspective* and *frame*. In order to highlight the ways in which disorders of thinking and language manifest themselves in schizophrenia, three areas where linguistics overlap with neuroscience and cognitive science in general were analyzed: metaphor, irony, and the coherence of conversations.

2.2 Metaphor

Vico (1744) considers that metaphor is an instrument of cognition that lies at the origin of language. Both in historical and contemporary use, it is understood and presented only as a rhetorical figure.[1] Traditionally, the following aspects of metaphor (Fig. 2.1) are emphasized as essential:

1. Nonliteral utterance emerging from literal, codified meaning
2. "Transferred"/figurative use: Exceptional/irregular word usage and deviation from the rule of usage (Kurz, 1997, p. 14)
3. Lack of comparison

---

[1] Aristoteles, Poetik, 21, 57b, 6, Aristoteles, Rhetorik, III, 10, 1410b, Borg (2004), Cacciari (1991, p. 3), Cappelen and Lepore (2005), Carston (2002), Eco (2005, p. 149–204); Ervas and Gola (2016), Genette (1972, pp. 21–40), Gensini (2004, pp. 35–38), Gibbs (2008), Kövecses (2000), Kövecses (2002), Kövecses (2005), Lakoff and Johnson (1980), Lo Piparo (2003), Lorusso (2005), Manetti (2005), Mortara Garavelli (1989, p. 163), Ortony (1975, pp. 45–53), Ortony (1979), Pragglejaz Group (2007, pp. 1–39), Richards (1936), Schmidt et al. (2007, pp. 273–294), Sperber and Wilson (1986), Stanley (2007), Stehen (2004, pp. 1295–1313), Travaglini (2009), Vico (1744, p. 283), Wilson and Sperber (2012).

P. Parisi, *A Phenomenological Interpretation of Schizophrenia*,
https://doi.org/10.1007/978-3-031-67860-8_2

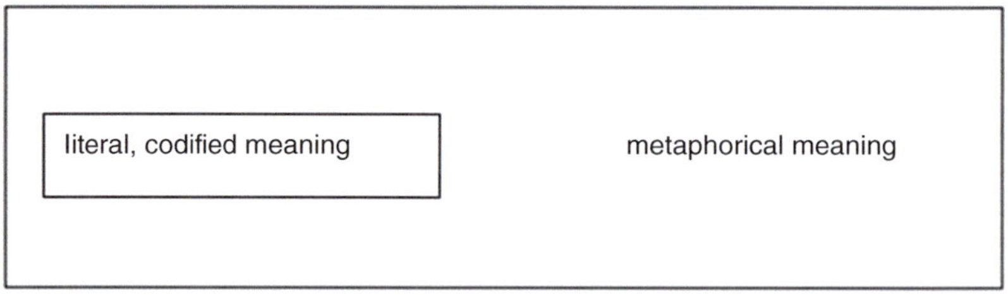

Fig. 2.1 Aspects of metaphor (own figure)

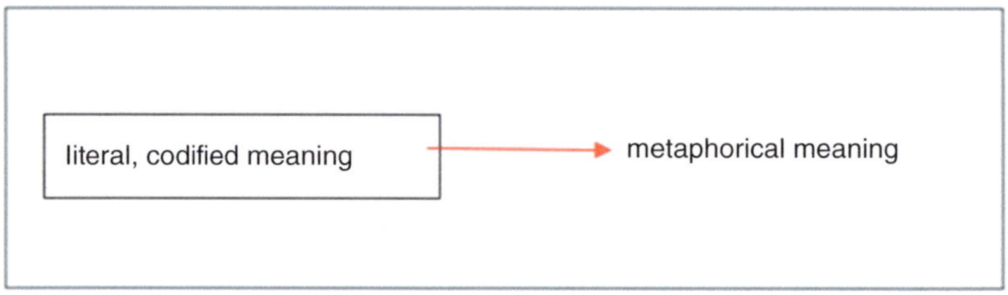

Fig. 2.2 Two semantic domains of metaphor (own figure)

Between the literal, codified meaning and the metaphorical meaning, there is a clear dividing line. In the terminology of this study, this metaphorical meaning lies outside an expected, codified *frame*. From this it can be concluded that, as far as the understanding of metaphorical expressions is concerned, this frame must be simultaneously recognized and extrapolated.

The word *metaphor*, from the ancient Greek verb *μεταφορέω*, indicates the crossing of a border, a boundary. "I carry elsewhere, transfer, transport." In this context, Umberto Eco observes that the word *μεταφορείς* can now be read by everyone on public transport traveling around the Greek peninsula (Eco, 2014).

For the present study, it is possible to stick to the demarcation suggested by the words *μετα-φορέω* and *transfer or carry over*, although there may be a continuum between regular and irregular word use.

The word *μεταφορέω* has the prefix *μετα*, similar to the German prefix *über-* (trans-). Therefore, the original literal meaning of the Greek word μεταφορέω means "to carry over."

Two semantic domains can be distinguished (Fig. 2.2):

1. The literal
2. The indirect or metaphorical

There is a disruption between these two areas that must be overcome in order to establish metaphorical meaning.

The arrow indicates the transcending of the conceptual frame that makes a metaphor possible. Without the frame that demarcates the literal meaning from the figurative one, one cannot form a metaphor, that is, one cannot perform a *metaphorizing operation*. The indispensable prerequisite for understanding any metaphor is that it can clearly represent the two levels of discourse—two levels that are distinct yet closely related.

What exactly do *signifier* and *signified* represent in the linguistic analysis of metaphors? What exactly can *metaphorical meaning* mean? That is, where does the arrow of metaphorical interpretation of a literal statement point to?

To answer these questions, it is important to bear in mind that most linguistic studies on metaphor and the possibilities of understanding metaphor date from about the second half of the 20th century, when the philosophers of *ideal language* failed to agree with the philosophers of *ordinary language*. The former sought a perfect, unambiguous ideal language. The latter focused their attention more on the use that speakers make of a language rather than on its ideal meaning. Philosophers of ideal language, i.e., philosophers of a positivist approach, include Gottlob Frege, Bertrand Russell, the Ludwig Wittgenstein of the *Tractatus Logico-Philosophicus* (the early Wittgenstein), and Alfred Tarski. Among philosophers of the ordinary language, the Wittgenstein of the *Philosophical Investigations* (the later Wittgenstein), John Austin, Gilbert Ryle, and Peter Strawson stand out. The later Wittgenstein, as opposed to the earlier one, denied the possibility of translating the language of speakers in real conversational contexts into the *ideal language*. The dichotomy between ideal and ordinary language was overcome by Paul Grice who made a distinction between the meaning of linguistic expressions and the use of linguistic expressions. The use of linguistic expression is directly related to the intention of speaker in a given context. In his work *Meaning* (1957, pp. 377–388), Grice distinguishes between natural and nonnatural meaning of a linguistic expression: The first meaning is independent of the speaker's intention, while the second is inseparable from it. For Grice, it is not only important what is said but also what is intended to be said. Grice's model of inference plunges those theories of meaning that understand language reductively according to the model of a code into a crisis. Based on the philosophical teaching of the later Wittgenstein, language opens up from assumed fixed meanings to use-dependent, context-sensitive meanings. The *con-text* is literally that which is *surrounding the text*. Thus, it is possible to understand what it means to get from the literal to the figurative or metaphorical meaning of a statement. The context provides a frame within which a metaphorical meaning must be developed. Grice's conception can be summarized in the following schema, which distinguishes three levels of meaning:

1. That which is linguistically encoded (the conventional meaning)
2. That which is said (the explicit meaning of the statement)
3. That which is implied (the implied meaning of the statement)

The current linguistic debate partly focuses on the question of what can be attributed to lexical, literal meanings and what contribution context makes to the constitution of meaning. The terms *literalism* and *contextualism* describe two standpoints in cognitive science: Contextualists believe that the pragmatics of language is also prevalent in what has traditionally been considered to belong to semantics. By way of contrast, for *contextualists*, the truth conditions of a statement are determined pragmatically and not semantically. Experimental pragmatics encompasses a huge number of studies in which metaphor is examined under the conditions of practical language use. For instance, the times and phases of the pragmatic processes involved in understanding metaphors are included in the analysis.

What has been the contribution of experimental pragmatics and linguistic metaphor research? The most important research in the linguistic field has been done on the understanding of metaphorical meaning: Does the understanding of literal or metaphorical meaning come first? The researchers who claim that the literal understanding of metaphor comes first belong to Grice's school of thought and describe this thesis as the *priority of the literal*. A metaphor like "You are the sun!" said to one's beloved, if taken literally, is blatantly false. however, the literalists argue that if the phrase "You are the sun!" is not to be taken literally, then it must be interpreted metaphorically. For these scholars, the understanding of the metaphorical meaning always happens in an indirect way and only after one has discarded the first literal understanding of the statement (Clark & Lucy, 1975, pp. 56–72). The hypothesis of the priority of the literal seems to be confirmed by behavioral studies showing that reading statements containing metaphors takes longer than reading literal statements (Bobrow & Bell, 1973, pp. 343–346; Gibbs, 1994; Gibbs, 2001, pp. 317–333; Janus & Bever, 1985, pp. 473–487).

In contrast to the studies of the literalists, however, other experiments have been conducted by contextualist-oriented scholars who do not see the necessity of an initial approach via the literal meaning in the interpretation of metaphor. The contextualists defend the thesis of the *direct access view* in which the implicit meaning of a metaphor is to be understood directly, without prior decoding of the literal meaning. Experimental studies that have used this approach have shown that the response times required to understand *phrasemes* (lexicalized fixed idioms) with metaphors are not always longer than the reaction times required to understand literal expressions (Gildea & Glucksberg, 1983, pp. 577–590; Glucksberg, 2001; Inhoff et al., 1984, pp. 558–567).

One point of agreement between literalists and contextualists on the approach to understanding metaphors can be explained as follows: Not all metaphors are the same, for some are *alive* and others are *dead*, i.e., lexicalized. Dead metaphors require no special imagination and are usually used by speakers directly in the metaphorical and therefore nonliteral meaning. Living metaphors are problematic, being relatively difficult to understand because they require both literal and figurative understanding. When Italians metaphorically say to someone "Sei un leone!" ("You are a lion," i.e., the person has great courage; in German, this is equivalent to the expression "einen Löwenmut haben" (to have a lion's courage)), they process it so immediately that the processing time to understand such a statement is no longer than for lexicalized expressions. This is an example of a dead or lexicalized metaphor that has entered widely into common usage. It is the opposite with living metaphors. To say that an important new discovery in biology is "the boson of biology" means that this discovery is as spectacular in biology as the discovery of the Higgs boson was in physics. Understanding this living metaphor is more difficult because it requires processing vast lexical, contextual, cultural, and encyclopedic information. In this case, access to the metaphorical and indirect meaning is mediated by a range of cultural and cognitive assumptions.

Linguistic research in the field of experimental pragmatics has initiated a line of research called *clinical pragmatics* (Cummings, 2014, 2017). Studies on the relationship between language and psychopathology have a long history. Having briefly addressed the meaning and ways of understanding metaphor, we are now prepared to continue our analysis in the psychopathological domain and, in particular, as regards the relationship between schizophrenia and metaphor. The basic question that we now need to address is how the concepts of frame and perspective change in individuals with schizophrenia. Two studies serve as paradigmatic examples of two different levels of impairment in the *framing*. One level is limited to a single sentence and the other to an entire text.

2.2.1 First Study

The first study describes and records an impairment of the *framing*-function, which manifests itself in an inability to understand metaphors. The study was conducted by Mossaheb and his colleagues at the University of Vienna (Mossaheb, 2014) and consists of several clinical studies carried out in the German language, with a focus on the comprehension of proverbs, as cases of metaphorical sentences. The study was carried out with 40 patients with schizophrenia and 43 non-schizophrenic subjects who were given a questionnaire containing 12 German proverbs. Some proverbs had to be paraphrased in different words, while for other proverbs the correct meaning had to be chosen from four possible alternatives: a) metaphorically correct, b) metaphorically incorrect, c) literally correct, and d) literally incorrect. The proverbs selected by the group of psychiatrists for the test were as follows:

1. Wir sitzen alle im gleichen Boot. (We are all in the same boat.)
2. Paul hat eine lange Leitung. (Paul is slow to catch on.)
3. Du bringst mich auf die Palme. (You are driving me up the wall.)
4. Ich lasse Sabine ein bisschen zappeln. (I have Sabine on the hook.)
5. Sie beißt nun in den sauren Apfel. (She is now biting the bullet.)
6. Barbara und Lisa geraten sich ständig in die Haare. (Barbara and Lisa always lock horns.)
7. Johanna hat die Katze aus dem Sack gelassen. (Johanna has let the cat out of the bag.)
8. Es streut Salz in ihre Wunde. (He rubs salt into her wound.)
9. Sie hat viel Staub aufgewirbelt. (She has risen a stink.)
10. Jetzt brennt ihm der Hut. (Literally: Now his hat is on fire. Meaning: To be in a mess; to be in a situation of urgency.)
11. Ich musste in letzter Zeit Vieles schlucken. (Literally: I had to swallow a lot lately. Meaning: I had to accept things without question or without expressing disagreement/I had to endure a lot lately.)

12. Ich rede anscheinend gegen eine Mauer. (I seem to be talking to a brick wall.)

Both non-schizophrenic subjects and patients with schizophrenia had to undergo several response tests of the following type:

1. Du bringst mich auf die Palme. (You are driving me up the wall.)
   (a) Du machst mich wütend. (You make me angry.)
   (b) Mir gefallen Palmen nicht so gut wie dir. (I don't like walls as much as you do.)
   (c) Ich helfe dir gerne. (I am happy to help you.)
   (d) Für dich klettere ich auf die Palme. (For you, I will climb up the wall.)
2. Ich musste in letzter Zeit viel schlucken. (See above: Literally: I had to swallow a lot lately.)
   (a) Ich musste in letzter Zeit viele Tabletten schlucken. (I had to swallow a lot of pills lately.)
   (b) Ich musste in letzter Zeit viel essen und trinken. (I had to eat and drink a lot lately.)
   (c) Ich musste in letzter Zeit viel ertragen. (I had to endure a lot lately.)
   (d) Ich musste in letzter Zeit viel lernen. (I had to learn a lot lately.)
3. Wir sitzen alle im gleichen Boot. (We are all in the same boat.)
   (a) Wir befinden uns im selben Boot. (We are in the same boat.)
   (b) Wir befinden uns in gleicher Lage und sind aufeinander angewiesen. (We are in the same situation and depend on each other.)
   (c) Wir müssen die Sache ausdiskutieren. (We have to talk this through.)
   (d) Wir kaufen uns zusammen ein Boot. (We buy a boat together.)

These three examples show how the tested subjects had to choose between metaphorical (true or false) and literal (true or false) meanings. Were there differences in the responses between patients with schizophrenia and non-schizophrenic subjects?

The authors of the study conclude:

> The aim of our study was to analyse potential differences between individuals with schizophrenia-spectrum disorders and healthy control subjects in their ability to recognise and paraphrase conventional metaphors. Our results clearly indicate impairments in patients' performance in all metaphor appreciation tasks used in this study with medium to large effect sizes. These findings confirm our hypotheses and are in line with previous studies that have shown deficits in figurative language comprehension in patients with schizophrenia compared to either psychiatric or non-psychiatric controls [...]. On a descriptive level, patients tended to interpret idiomatic expressions more often on a literal level. Regarding multiple-choice as well as paraphrastic answers in conventional metaphor comprehension, significant group differences were found (multiple choice answers: t (81) = 4.62 $\leq$ 0.0001, $r = 0.21$; paraphrastic answers: t (81) = 3.55, $p \leq 0.0001$, $r = 0.37$) with lower comprehension of metaphors in patients with schizophrenia and schizoaffective disorders. (Mossaheb, 2014, p. 931)

If we intend to create a schema in order to illustrate the deficit in the understanding of metaphor, we can, again, use the notion of the frame.

The deficit identified by Mossaheb and his colleagues mainly concerns the inability, which is frequently observed in individuals with schizophrenia, to make the transition of understanding a sentence from the literal level to the metaphorical level (Fig. 2.3). Patients with schizophrenia do not have the ability to focus on the frame that separates the actual from the figurative meaning of a sentence, statement, or proverb; they are unable to properly understand the meaning of an expression in the context of lived life. There are habitual, lexicalized metaphors and innovative metaphors. Patients with schizophrenia often have problems even with comprehending lexicalized metaphors. Unfortunately, the studies on this aspect are not very nuanced. This much can be said: Patients with schizophrenia obviously stay within the frame of what they have once learned, without attempting to adapt their interpretations to the lifeworld and the world of common experience.

2.2.2 Second Study

What happens when the focus of the investigation is shifted from the meaning of a single sentence (such as a proverb) to that of a whole metaphorical text? If the aim is to understand how speakers integrate the linguistic information of a single sentence into a wider context (such as language or background knowledge), then new experimental designs need to be developed that are able to take into account processes that go in their scope beyond the single sentence.

Towards the end of the 1990s, a research field was established that focused on *ERPs* (event-related potentials) measured by means of EEG. Some of these studies were conducted specifically on the topic of metaphor (Arzouan et al., 2007; Bambini, 2017; De Grauwe, 2010; Lai et al., 2009; Pynte, 1996; Tartter et al., 2002). In 1980, Kutas and Hillyard (1980, pp. 203–205) analyzed the brain's response by comparing sentences such as:

(a) John has eaten bread with *socks*.
(b) John has eaten bread with *honey*.

The sentences were presented word by word. In the case of the semantic anomaly, the EEG showed a negative wave of 400 milliseconds. The response was called *N400* (*N* = negative polarity; *400* = time delay). The researchers interpreted these

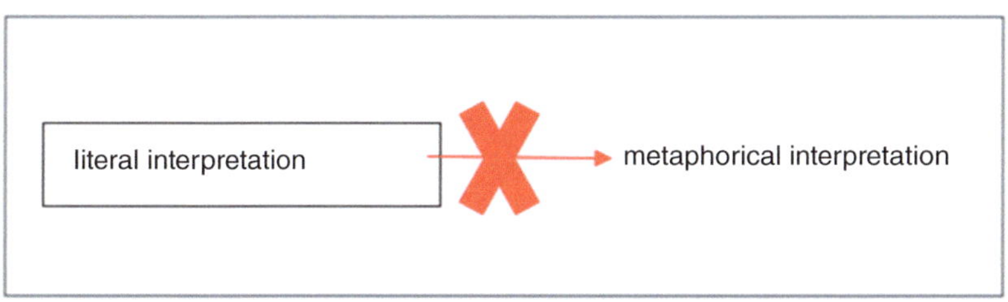

Fig. 2.3 Graph for a common deficit in patients with schizophrenia (own figure)

data as the effect that occurs during the semantic processing of a word that is unexpected in its context. This experiment was repeated by other researchers who also observed this response in other languages and other situations.

About 20 years after Kutas' and Hillyard's experiment, another experiment was conducted in which the focus shifted from a single sentence to a larger context into which a sentence was inserted (Van Berkum et al., 1999, pp. 657–671). The experiment consisted of examining the response of the N400 to the variation of a word that was coherent or incoherent with the general context. This text was presented to the subjects:

> As agreed upon, Jane was to wake her sister and her brother at five o'clock in the morning. But the sister had already washed herself, and the brother had even got dressed. Jane told the brother that he was exceptionally … (Van Berkum et al., 1999, p. 659.).

(a) …slow
(b) …fast

The analysis of the ERPs showed that the unexpected word (slow) elicited a N400, while the other word (fast) did not.

What happens when an unexpected sentence is integrated into an otherwise consistent text? This question was examined by means of an experiment conducted a few years later by Nieuwland and Van Berkum (Nieuwland & Van Berkum, 2006, pp. 1098–1111). The research participants were asked to read the following sentences:

(a) The peanut was *salted.*
(b) The peanut was *in love.*

Again, the incoherent sentence (b) evoked a N400 response. The adjective *in love* is unusual in the semantic frame formed by the word *peanut*. However, everything changes when the same sentence is inserted into a text that sets a different frame in which the peanut behaves like an animated being:

> A woman saw a dancing peanut who had a big smile on his face. The peanut was singing about a girl he had just met. And judging from the song, the peanut was totally crazy about her. The woman thought it was really cute to see the peanut singing and dancing like that. (Nieuwland & Van Berkum, 2006, p. 1106)

If we now ask respondents to reread the sentence "The peanut was salted/in love" in view of the passage above, the direction of the N400 effect reverses. This experiment shows that N400 is sensitive to expectations set by the frame. The frames set by the context are so strong that they take precedence over the frames set by the individual words. The frame of the whole speech is relevant for the perception of coherence.

Boudewyn and his colleagues built on this experiment (Boudewyn et al., 2017, pp. 262–273) by subjecting patients with schizophrenia to an ERP analysis while they were reading the following text:

> A lucky peanut had a big smile on his face. The peanut was amazed about his good fortune. Just now he had won the jackpot of two million dollars. The peanut was *elated/salted* and who could blame him. (Boudewyn et al., 2017, p. 37)

The underlying hypothesis was that in contrast to non-schizophrenic individuals in the control group, patients with schizophrenia have more difficulties integrating information from the context in order to complete the sentence by selecting the appropriate adjective *elated*. In both groups, the amplitude of N400 was higher for the contextually inappropriate word *salted* than for the more coherent word *elated*. However, the effect of N400 is smaller in patients with schizophrenia than in the control group. This means that the adjective *salted* did not seem as inappropriate to the individuals with schizophrenia as it did to the non-schizophrenic subjects. Integrating information from the context, which has been statistically proven by the authors, is apparently more difficult for patients with schizophrenia than for non-schizophrenic individuals.

Boudewyn's experiment shows how fundamental the context is for a meaningful interpretation of the sentence (Fig. 2.4). In this case, it is about the application of a double frame. In Mossaheb's experiment, patients with schizophrenia had difficulties distinguishing the literal from the metaphorical meaning of a sentence (proverb). In Boudewyn's experiment, the problem is the metaphorical interpretation of a sentence that has no meaning in itself. To say that a peanut is elated makes no sense. This statement can only become coherent if it is justified in a context in which the (literally meaningless) sentence is inserted.

Both types of impairments in the use and understanding of metaphors have in common the recognition and intelligent management of interpretive frames and the ability to shift between different perspectives and viewpoints. Thomas Fuchs, psychiatrist and philosopher at Heidelberg University, emphasizes this crucial aspect in the understanding of metaphors in patients with schizophrenia: They tend to interpret metaphors only in the literal sense, thus gaining only a concrete interpretation

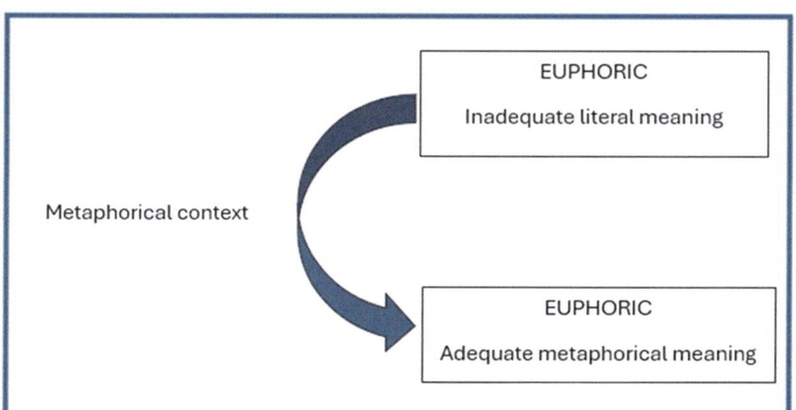

Fig. 2.4 Graph of the metaphorical understanding in Boudewyn's experiment (own figure)

of the sentence. *Concretism* means the tendency towards concrete (literal) rather than metaphorical (figurative) interpretation. Fuchs also takes up the idea of the frame as a separating element between the literal and the figurative:

> A metaphor combines two terms or objects: Usually, the one signifies a concrete object of bodily experience, while the other means the abstract term which shows some kind of analogy to the first. Thus, we speak of a 'grain of truth', as if truth could be found in the soil, or of the 'evening of life' as if life could have a sunset. The metaphor oscillates between two meanings of frameworks of reference which have both to be held present in order to understand the metaphor's 'as-if'. (Fuchs, 2017a, p. 87 f.)

Similar to the approach presented in this book, Fuchs also combines frame and perspective to explain the difference in metaphorical thinking between non-schizophrenic individuals and individuals with schizophrenia:

> To keep up the difference between both levels of meaning is part of perspectival flexibility. Schizophrenia patients, however, may be unable to maintain this 'as-if' and the two levels of meaning collapse into one. (Fuchs, 2017b, p. 87 f.)

Fuchs provides examples to prove that in the thinking of individuals with schizophrenia, expressions used metaphorically are understood concretely, for instance, the German expressions "Das ist Gold wert" (that is worth its weight in gold) or "schmutzige Gedanken" (dirty thoughts). A similar phenomenon is the inability of patients with schizophrenia to understand the metaphorical meaning of proverbs, as the following examples show:

> (a) Psychiatrist: "Too many cooks spoil the broth."
> Patient's explanation: "Well, if a cook is responsible for the kitchen, one should leave it to them, otherwise the dinner will be spoiled."
> (b) Psychiatrist: "One should strike while the iron is hot."
> Patient: "I would say, heat makes the iron soft, so you can better forge or shape it."
> Obviously, the abstract explanation on the track of the "as-if" requires a higher cognitive effort than just sticking to the level of the literal. Again, the double intention inherent in the use of proverbs is lost, and the concrete and metaphorical level collapse into one. The explanation of proverbs may therefore be used as a diagnostic marker for schizophrenia. (Fuchs, 2017a, p. 87 f.)

The phenomenon of typical concretism in schizophrenia[2] can therefore rightly be interpreted as the inability to make appropriate use of both interpretive frames and meaning perspectives.[3]

---

[2] Chapman (1960, pp. 412–416), Holm-Hadulla (1982, pp. 524–529), Holm-Hadulla and Haug (1984, pp. 496–503), Holm-Hadulla (1988, pp. 1–7), Kasanin (1944), Rapp et al. (2018, pp. 1–11), Rossetti et al. (2018, pp. 1–15), Strobl and Resch (1988, pp. 99–102), Thoma and Daum (2006, pp. 1182–1205).

[3] Brune and Bodenstein (2005, pp. 233–239), Gavilán Ibáñey and García-Albea Ristol (2011, pp. 54–69), Green (2012, pp. 854–864), Langdon et al. (2002, pp. 68–104), Mitchley (1998, pp. 127–138), Rapp et al. (2014).

2.3 Irony

Two aspects are of primary importance for a valid interpretation of any ironic conversation:

1. Irony presupposes a disagreement between an objective factual situation and a statement that presents or evaluates this situation from a counterfactual perspective.
2. Without a common recognition of the facts by the interlocutors, the ironic perspective of interpretation cannot be adopted. "Irony as a thought *tropus* [...] consists [...] in the replacement of the intended thought by an alternative thought." (Lausberg, 1949, p. 237; source in German)

As regards irony, the process of recognition is complicated because three factors have to be considered simultaneously: the state of things (*the context*), the meaning of the statement (*the text*), and the speaker's intentions (the *speaker's perspective*). These intentions (*the illocutionary components* of a speech) are often very clearly co-formulated, while irony signals (intonation, facial expression, gestures) may well be missing.

The classic and simplest example of an ironic statement is the exclamation "What a beautiful day!" during a heavy thunderstorm that may have ruined the weekend outing or picnic with family and friends. This example contains all the elements mentioned above (Fig. 2.5).

The understanding of irony presupposes that the perspectives of the interlocutors have shared agreement on the facts.

Studies in experimental psychology and linguistic pragmatics have also shown that understanding irony is more difficult and complex than understanding metaphors, for instance (Marchetti et al., 2007). The difficulties of comprehending irony

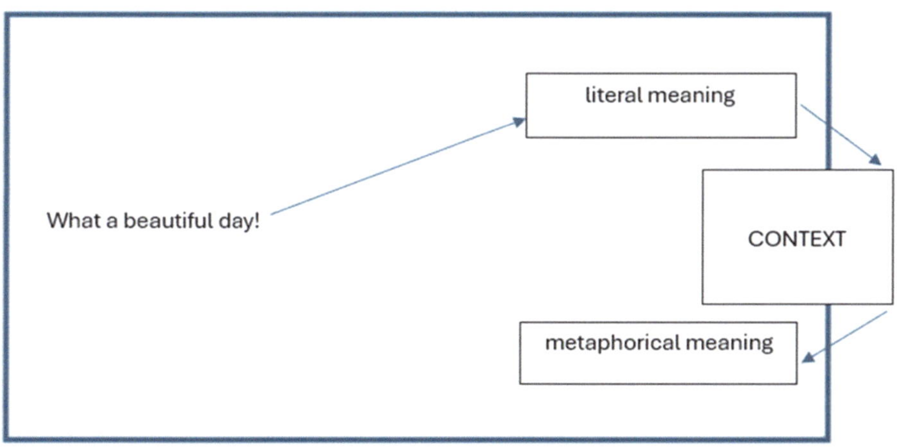

Fig. 2.5 Graph showing the comprehension of an example of an ironic statement (own figure)

can be clearly illustrated by the experiments conducted in the context of the *theory of mind.*

The theory of mind describes the capacity of individuals to ascribe mental states to themselves and to others and to predict their behavior on the basis of these states (Premack & Woodruff, 1978).

According to Astington, Harris, and Olson, the *theory of mind encompasses*:

1. The ability to recognize oneself and others as thinking beings
2. The ability to recognize mental states (intentions, desires, beliefs) in oneself and others as a different capacity, rather than simply "experiencing" these states
3. The ability to refer explicitly to one's own and others' minds and to use these concepts to explain and predict what one can do or say oneself or what others can do or say

The theory of mind is a specific field of reflection within the cognitive sciences and was developed within the framework of an experimental paradigm known as the *false belief test* (Wimmer & Perner, 1983, pp. 103–128).

Figure 2.6 is the best-known version of this test (Baron-Cohen et al., 1985, pp. 37–46).

Sally and Anne are the protagonists of this illustration. Sally has a basket and Anne has a box. Sally has a marble and puts it in her basket. Then she goes away. While Sally is away, Anne takes Sally's marble out of the basket and puts it in her box. Sally comes back and wants to play with her marble. At this point, the children taking the test are asked where they would look for the marble if they were Sally. The correct answer is, of course, in the basket. Children under 4 years of age do not pass this test. They cannot distinguish the actual situation from what they believe is the situation yet, i.e., they cannot consider what others may not have seen. The results of this experiment have been experimentally repeated many times (Wellman et al., 2001, pp. 655–684). In recent years, it has been demonstrated that children under the age of 2 are able to pass nonverbal false belief tests (Baillargeon et al., 2010, pp. 110–118; Onishi & Baillargeon, 2005, pp. 255–258).

In recent research, children aged 12 months were placed in different situations where they observed an adult looking for an object that had fallen from a shelf. In these situations, the child would indicate by means of gestures where the object being searched for was located, if the adult had not seen the object fall. However, no information was provided by the children if the adult had observed the scene (Liszkowski et al., 2008, pp. 732–739).

The false belief test explains what it means to be able to understand the intentions of others. To understand irony, one must also know the context of an utterance. In an ironic speech act, "A" can mean "Not A." The context is crucial for understanding the meaning of a sentence and thus the speaker's intention (Basnáková, 2013, pp. 2572–2578). As Valentina Bambini says, irony is the prototypical case of a distance between meaning and opinion (Bambini, 2017, pp. 57–58).

In summary, the premises of irony are as follows:

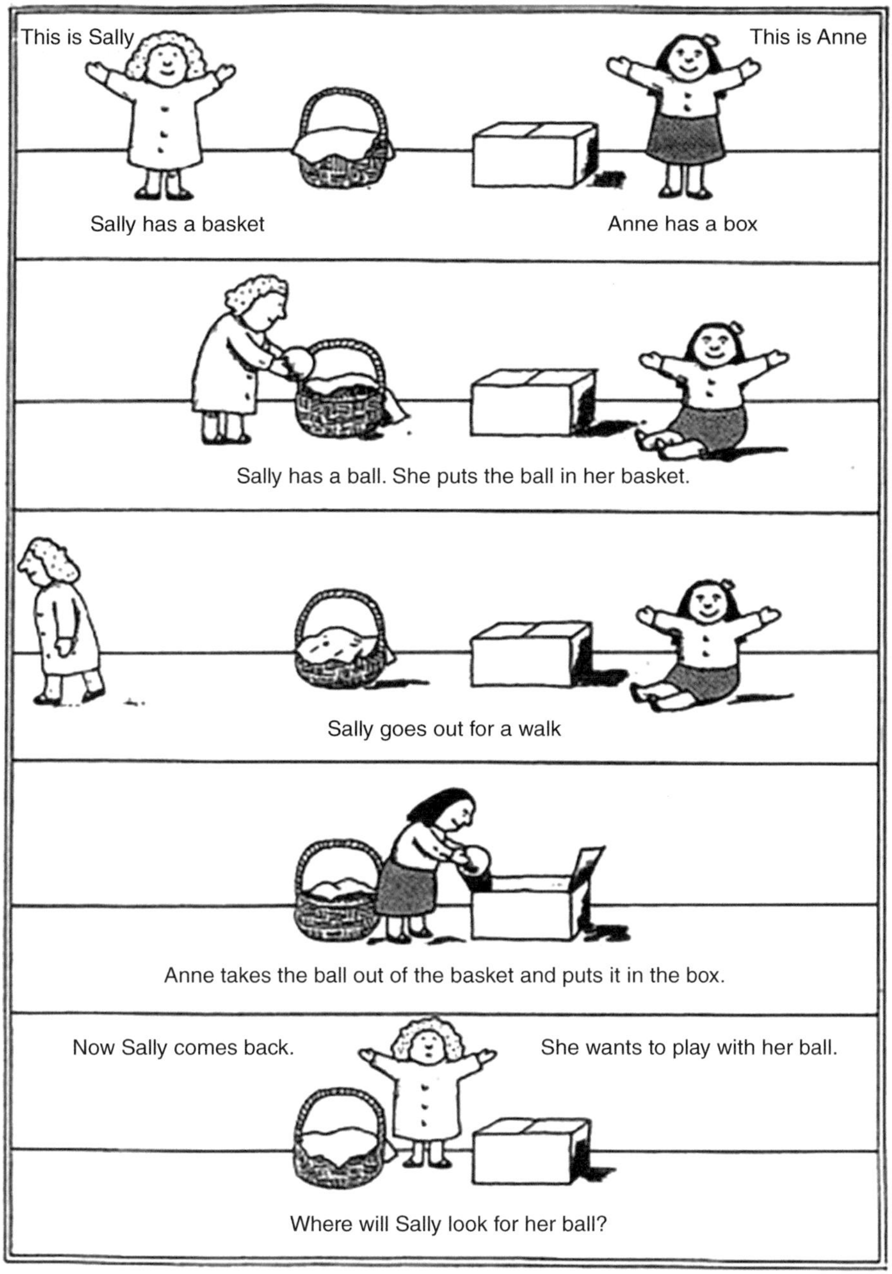

Fig. 2.6 False belief test (Baron-Cohen et al., 1985, p. 41)

(a) The grasping of one's own thinking subjectivity and the recognition of other thinking subjectivities (as explained by the *theory of mind*)
(b) The certainty of an objective fact
(c) The understanding of contextual and illocutionary elements

Clearly, an awareness of perspectives and frames is fundamental to understanding irony.

The question that now arises is: How do patients with schizophrenia react to irony? According to the premises outlined, one expects serious impairments.

Over the last 30 years, several studies have been conducted with patients with schizophrenia in order to assess their abilities with regard to the *theory of mind*, first by Frith (1992), Frith and Corcoran (1996, pp. 521–530), Doody (1998, pp. 397–405), and later by Langdon (1997, pp. 167–193), Langdon (2001, pp. 81–108), Langdon (2002, pp. 1273–1284). Mazza pointed out that patients with chronic schizophrenia and normal IQ scores reached poorer false belief test scores than control subjects (Mazza, 2001, pp. 299–308). Similar results were also found by Brüne (2003, pp. 57–64).

To understand irony, one must understand the thoughts and intentions of the other, as the *second-order theory of mind* explains. Within a *frame theory,* one can speak of double framing:

> Every conversation with others implies a continuous oscillation between my central, embodied perspective and the decentered or virtual perspective from which I am aware of the other as being aware of me. I have to put my body-centered existence into brackets and for a moment pretend to be in the other's place. However, in order not to lose myself in this oscillation, it is also necessary to keep up the difference between the embodied and the virtual perspective. It is this dialectical tension of the eccentric position that the schizophrenic patient cannot maintain anymore. The perspectives of self and other are confused instead of being integrated from the eccentric position, resulting in a sense of being invaded and overpowered by the other. (Fuchs, 2017b, p. 89)

The impaired understanding of irony in persons with schizophrenia is therefore the result of the inability to deal flexibly with linguistic and intentional perspectives and frames of situation and meaning.

2.4 Coherence and Cohesion

Schizophrenic speech has also often been said to lack consistency. Michael Halliday and Ruqaiya Hasan have explored the semantic and etymological connection between the English terms *text* and *texture* (Halliday & Hasan, 1976). Any coherent and cohesive text represents a unified texture. Linguistic research in recent decades has broadened the study of language from sentence to text. The definition of *cohesion* by Rochester and Martin (1979) is not far from the idea of a framework of meaning that a text represents when it forms a thematic unit as a whole:

The concept of cohesion is used to refer to the semantic relations within a text that make it a unit. Cohesion is said to occur where the interpretation of some element in the discourse is dependent on another element. The one presumes the other, in the sense that the one cannot be effectively understood except by recourse to the other. For example, in

1. There was a donkey about to cross a river.
   It was loaded with bags of salt.

It is clear that the second sentence refers back to a donkey in the first sentence. The referential relation between the two elements gives cohesion to the two sentences so that we interpret them as part of the same text. Texture is provided not by the elements themselves but by the cohesive relations that exist between them. The cohesion would not be effected by presence of the referring item *it*, alone. To give a sense of unity to the sentences, both the referring item and its referent must be present. As another example of a different sort of meaning relation which contributes to texture, consider the following:

2. Did I hurt your feelings?
   – I didn't mean to*.

Here, the second sentence coheres by virtue of the missing elements—I didn't mean to (hurt your feelings)—but, again, the *pair* of elements is needed to effect a bond. (Rochester & Martin, 1979, p. 74)

Within a speech or text, there are grammatical and conceptual links which give the text or the speech unity. These connections make it possible to link the sentences together and make them coherent within the common framework of the conversation. Rochester and Martin, who have written a (now classical) book on the language of individuals with schizophrenia, list five forms of cohesive devices used in speeches or texts:

Reference:

1. Pronominal: We met Joy Adamson and had dinner with *her* in Nairobi.
2. Demonstrative: We went to *a hostel* and oh *that* was a dreadful place.
3. Comparative: *Six guys* approached me. The *last* guy pulled a knife on me in the park.

Substitution:

1. Nominal: The oldest girl is 25 and the next *one's* 22.
2. Verbal: Eastern people *take it seriously*, at least some of them *do*.
3. Causal: *I'm making it worse for myself.* I would think *so*.

Ellipsis:

1. Nominal: He's got *energy* too. He's got a lot more Ø than I do.
2. Verbal: I could go to university all my life, Ø keep going to school.
3. Causal: Have you ever been to Israel? - No, my brother has Ø.*

Conjunction:

1. Additive: I read a book in the past few days *and* I like it.
2. Adversative: They started out to England *but* got captured on the way.
3. Causal: It was a beautiful tree, *so* I left it alone.
4. Temporal: My mother was in Ireland. *Then* she came over here.
5. Continuative: What kind of degree? – *Well*, in one of the professions.

Lexical:

1. Same root: Mother needs *independence*. She was always *dependent* on my father.
2. Synonym: *I got angry* at M., but I don't often *get mad*.
3. Superordinate: I love catching *fish*. I caught a *bass* last time.
4. General item: The *plane* hit some air pockets and the *bloody thing* went up and down (Rochester & Martin, 1979, p. 77).

Schizophrenic speech often shows an impairment in dealing with cohesion and coherence. This impairment manifests itself in different ways. Sometimes the answer to a question may seem tangential to the question asked. Other times, the subject of the conversation is lost sight of, which is a classical symptom of derailment. Difficulties in handling grammatical rules can also be observed.

Christopher Frith, referring to Andreasen's seminal studies (Andreasen, 1979, pp. 1325–1330), provides a list of the forms in which schizophrenic speech may appear deviant and the frequency with which these forms occur (Frith, 1992, p. 80):

1. Poverty of speech (29%)
2. Poverty of content of speech (40%)
3. Tangentiality (36%)
4. Derailment (56%)
5. Incoherence (16%)
6. Illogicality (27%)
7. Loss of goal (44%)
8. Perseveration (24%)
9. Self-reference (13%)

Adornetti generally states that schizophrenic speech is often disorganized and shows a lack formal thought (Adornetti, 2018, p. 125). In recent years, studies have been conducted to analyze the impairment of syntactic abilities in individuals with schizophrenia.[4] These studies have shown that schizophrenic speech is character-

[4] Ceccherini-Nelli and Crow (2003, pp. 233–240), Chen (1996, pp. 4–13), Condray and Steinhauer (2003, pp. 87–88), Covington (2005, pp. 85–98), De Lisi (1997, pp. 255–271), De Lisi (2001, pp. 481–496), Fraser (1986, pp. 275–278), Kircher (2005, pp. 209–214), Morice and Ingram (1982, pp. 11–21), Morice and McNicol (1985, pp. 567–580), Morice and McNicol (1986, pp. 239–251).

ized by marked syntactic simplifications. Other studies demonstrate a relationship between syntactic simplification and negative symptoms (Thomas et al., 1987, pp. 144–151; Thomas et al., 1990, pp. 204–210) and also between reduced syntactic complexity and worsening of the clinical conditions of patients with chronic schizophrenia (Thomas et al., 1990; King et al., 1990, pp. 211–215). Syntax impairment, as has already been observed by Rochester and Martin, corresponds to impairment of cohesion, which has also been demonstrated in recent studies by Docherty et al. (1996, 2003).

A group of researchers from the University of Verona led by Perlini (2012, pp. 363–376) conducted a study with 90 participants: 30 patients with schizophrenia, 30 patients with a bipolar disorder, and 30 healthy subjects. The results of the study confirm that individuals with schizophrenia have problems with both linguistic microstructures (at the grammatical level) and macrostructures (at the textual level). Perlini and colleagues report:

> We found significant difficulties in narrative production and syntactic comprehension in patients with schizophrenia. [...] As for narrative production, compared with the group of healthy control participants, schizophrenia patients produced speech samples with a normal amount of words, but with reduced speech rates, shorter utterances, a greater amount of paragrammatic errors, and lower levels of syntactic complexity. [...] Patients with schizophrenia had difficulties in establishing the semantic connectivity across contiguous and long-distant sentences (local and global coherence, respectively). (Perlini et al., 2012, pp. 372–373)

Conversations that took place in a Finnish research center between a psychiatrist and a 26-year-old patient with schizophrenia can illustrate the abovementioned observations. The conversations were video-recorded and then transcribed in the university's linguistics department. Below we look at two dialogues (Hella et al., 2013, pp. 320–328).

The first dialogue is a paradigmatic example of a tangential conversation (*round-about talk*; in German: *Danebenreden*) and is characterized by a gradual radial expansion of the topic.

Text 1:

Doctor: Has anybody else ever tried to harm you or tried to lead you to any kind of trouble?

Patient (1): Well, I have not thought about that ... but not (they have not led) me ... I have seen harm done and stuff, but people, those guys, let me be physically and mentally on my own...

Doctor: Have you ever felt you would be especially important or that you would have abilities that no one else has?

Patient (2): Well, it's only that my name is John [altered], which happens to be the kind that others are laughing at. They are laughing right to my face, and then...

Doctor: Why would they laugh at the name John?

Patient (3): Well, in some way that John that you

har-har.

Doctor: What does John mean?

Patient (4): Well I don't know John (aborted sentence) probably ... it refers to me and that a bit har-har and so on.

Doctor: I can't quite understand. Can you tell what it is ...

Patient (5): Then on the other hand...

Doctor: Uh-huh.

Patient (6): (shifting abruptly to his family name) ... there are those X-ers (X-er referring to people from area X, like New Yorker. X-er used here is also patient's family name) from Y (province capital) but yeah. As a joke, I kind of imagine that it (obscure, which name/location?) is a kind of sacred relic that I should not be teased for that (laughs).

Doctor: Do you mean that ...

Patient (7): Yeah.

Doctor: ... that your name is a relic.

Patient (8): Or my family name X-er is one, since I am one (i.e., an inhabitant of province X bearing the province name).

Doctor: Yeah, what does it mean ...

Patient (9): Well...

Doctor: ... that it is a relic.

Patient (10): Well, it occurs to me all the time that X is the town (literally: municipality) (erroneous statement, confusion of province and hometown names). It's definitely the town that is called X (erroneous statement repeated with emphasis) which is always seen on the (television) news ... rolling (makes rolling gestures with arms)

Doctor: Yeah.

Patient (11): X, yes. (yawning) Well, I also do have other names.

Doctor: What names?

Patient (12): I'd rather be some Marko, damn it, if I could myself decide upon taking a name.

Doctor: Why would you change your name?

Patient (13): Well, I don't know. It only occurred to me that it could be cool to be Marko, if not anything else, damn it. (Hella et al., 2013, pp. 320–328)

The dialogue represents a tangential patient response (2) and an abnormal extension of semantic associations. As noted by Ditman and Kuperberg, the derailment of the conversation makes the construction of a coherent holistic image, a quintessence of the conversation impossible (Ditman & Kuperberg, 2010, pp. 254–269; Ditman et al., 2011, pp. 245–258; Kuperberg et al., 2010, pp. 66–76). It is interesting how these authors have taken up the metaphor of the image as a holistic construction to show the global and coherent structure of a conversation.

Text 1 shows how the patient verbalizes irrelevant thought associations resulting from a semantic hyperactivation of the thoughts dealt with during the dialogue.

The second dialogue, on the other hand, is a clear example of a disorganized conversation which is characterized by a lack of linear organization of the topic and shows confusing and irrelevant references. It can be observed how the patient loses sight of the main topic of the conversation and is unable to follow the intended purpose of the dialogue. The sentences are juxtaposed and show little cohesion. The patient is not able to integrate the different contents of his statements into a unified structure of meaning.

Text 2:

Patient (116): I've been thinking about those that ... going to work I'm always thinking about. Then some people, well they are stars and the like, they play soccer, and we then watch, or they watch it and such like that.

Doctor: Yes, who are watching?

Patient (117): Trades/professions I kind of think about.

Doctor: Uh-huh.

Patient (118): They are a bit like a group of their own and such. They are jobless.

Doctor: Uh-uh, who are you talking about now?

Patient (119): Well, I'm thinking about these kinds of things. My father works at the city water works. Workers come to my mind sometimes.

Doctor: Yeah.

Patient (120): That's it. Well, that I would want to be a bit better educated, but I am not. Then I am not extremely clever, perhaps. In a way that sometimes, well yes, I do watch something. A group of people can come up with wise things but...things are not like that now.

Doctor: Yes. What...

Patient (121) (yawning) Well, I do have a trade school diploma. (Hella et al., 2013, pp. 320–328)

The metaphor of the frame as an element of cohesion and unity in a conversation was used by a group of researchers to describe the linguistic and pragmatic deficits in 37 patients with schizophrenia (Tavano, 2008). The conclusion of the study conducted by Tavano is in line with previous findings:

> In the narrative, where a subject's speech is guided by an ordered set of pictures, patients produced fewer words and propositions that healthy controls. Furthermore, they tended to repeat the words they had initially selected throughout the story, thereby yielding a significant lower lexical diversity index than controls. [...] In the conversational task, patients and healthy controls displayed similar lexical abilities, but they differed with respect to the frequency of complex syntactic clauses, which is significantly lower for patients. Preserved syntactic abilities are required in online utterance planning. It is likely that in our patients a reduced access to syntactic diversity resulted in structurally simpler utterances. Syntactic comprehension was also significantly more impaired in patients than in healthy controls, and such difference seems to be due to specifically syntactic errors. [...] We take this result to suggest that the linguistic impairment in schizophrenia specifically involves a reduced access to *structural syntactic frames.* (Tavano, 2008, p. 59)

In summary, one can say that many disorders of schizophrenic thinking and schizophrenic conversation show an impairment of the frame. It manifests itself, for instance, in the disability to focus on a particular topic.

The subject of the conversation is, so to speak, the perspectival vanishing point, i.e., the point to which all the elements of a composition should converge. If the perspective vanishing point is not present, the elements of the composition remain isolated.

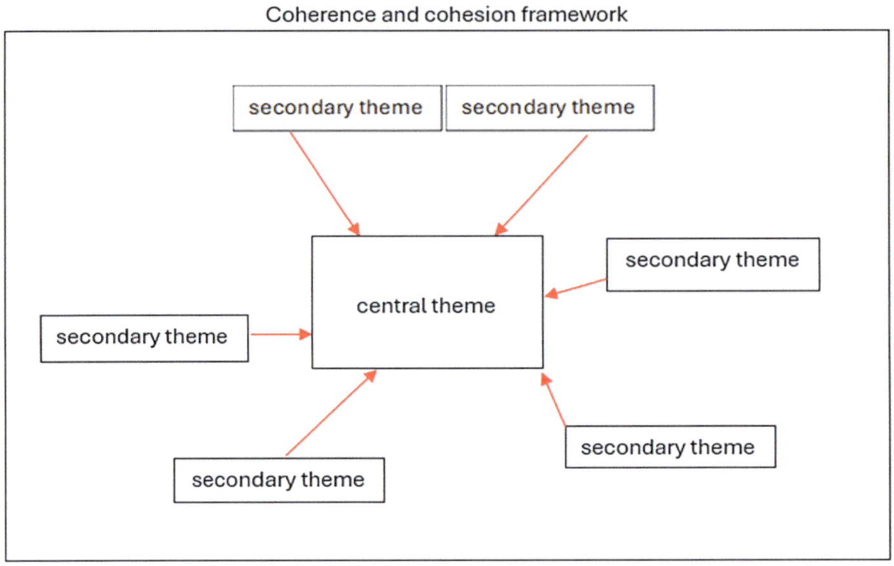

Fig. 2.7 Graph of the coherence and cohesion framework: the frame organizes central and secondary themes (own figure)

The terms *coherence* and *cohesion* have the prefix *co-* that comes from the Latin *cum and* means *together or with*. Coherence and cohesion in a speech only exist when all elements of it contribute to the formation of an overall picture.

At the sentence level, coherence is created by syntax. This is actually the original meaning of the word *syntax*. The Greek term *Σύνταξις* means *association* or *organization* and derives from the Greek prefix *σύν*, which has the same meaning as the Latin *cum* and the Greek term *τάξις*, which means *comprehensive order.*

Therefore, a sentence and a conversation can be depicted as a perspectival composition in which the central theme of the conversation is the vanishing point, and the frame delineates the area in which the various elements and different aspects of a given theme are coherently and cohesively located (Fig. 2.7). This is precisely what is often impaired in schizophrenia.

2.5 Summary

Individuals with schizophrenia show typical speech disorders. They have, for instance, difficulties understanding metaphors, especially those that are not lexicalized, and ironic speech. In addition, impairments in the ability to structure and organize a conversation coherently can be observed. These speech disorders, which are quite diverse, can result from a deficit in the ability to integrate the different elements of a conversation into a coherent frame. The absence or impairment of the frame leads to an impairment of the integration of language components. As a result, there is grammatical and conceptual *loosenesses* within texts. The frame is the element that both distinguishes and holds together text and context: If the frame is missing, it is difficult or impossible to understand both ironic and metaphorical speech. The loss of the frame also implies a loss of perspective. Associated with this is the loss of purposefulness and of the logical structure of the conversation. The *perspective* is also highly relevant for understanding irony. In order to understand the irony of an expression, it is necessary to understand both the linguistic text in its context and the perspective of the interlocutor. Thus, the concepts of frame and perspective give us the possibility to grasp different linguistic disorders in a unified hermeneutic paradigm.

3 Analysis of Social Behavior

3.1 Introduction

This chapter will present the micro-social behavior of patients with schizophrenia. Microsociology is the branch of sociology that emerged from the pioneering studies of Erving Goffman. Microsociology focuses on the study of social interaction in small human groups consisting of two or more people. In recent decades, microsociology has shed light on the importance of nonverbal communication; proxemics, i.e., the physical distance between speakers during a dialogue; gestures; facial expressions; and other forms of human interaction. In this chapter, specific problems that patients with schizophrenia have with the perception of human interactions involving the face and body are described in a phenomenological approach.

3.2 Face

What would our daily lives be like were we unable to understand or interpret emotions through people's facial expressions? By looking at a person's face, we can already grasp much of the emotional atmosphere that dominates a space or a particular situation. Such intuitive knowledge is also reflected in everyday language. The expression "love at first sight," for instance, means the simultaneous recognition of the other person's and one's own emotions from the moment of meeting. The Italian expression "Gli occhi dei padri, la legge dei figli" (The eyes of the fathers, the law of the children) ascribes not only an emotional but also a moral importance to the gaze: Children recognize from the face, the expression, and the eyes of their parents whether their behavior is appropriate or not, whether what they do at a particular moment pleases the parents or not. They communicate all this without speaking, recognizing, and understanding in the very short time in which their eyes meet their parents' emotions. If we consider too the Italian idiom "Gli occhi sono lo specchio dell' anima" (the eyes are the mirror of the soul), we are also here reminded

P. Parisi, *A Phenomenological Interpretation of Schizophrenia*,
https://doi.org/10.1007/978-3-031-67860-8_3

of the importance of nonverbal communication. We create an emotional atmosphere through our mere presence, our facial features, and our way of looking.

Things that are normally experienced naturally and spontaneously in everyday life are severely impaired in schizophrenia. Understanding the emotions of others quickly and skillfully is important for a healthy social life. Many researchers have recently found serious deficits in facial and emotional perception in patients with schizophrenia. Some of the studies are very cleverly designed, for example, one of the studies reveals that individuals with schizophrenia recognize facial expressions better in black and white photographs than in color. In this study, the photographs presented to the subjects in the study showed neutral or sad facial expressions (Silver & Bilker, 2015, pp. 438–455).

It has been shown that the inability to read emotions in facial expressions affects the well-being in social relationships.[1]

The incomplete exploration of other faces is one of the causes why individuals with schizophrenia have difficulties in adequately understanding the emotions of others. While non-schizophrenic individuals predominantly focus on the salient features of the face (eyes, nose, and mouth), individuals with schizophrenia, as some eye tracking studies show, concentrate on less significant areas such as the cheeks and chin. Thus, individuals with schizophrenia scan the faces of other persons in a limited way (Loughland et al., 2002, pp. 159–170; Phillips & David, 1998, pp. 235–245), which is why the recognition of emotions such as happiness, sadness, or anger is impaired.[2] Some researchers have even suggested that eye tracking facial scans showing unusual results could be used as markers for schizophrenia (Loughland et al., 2004, pp. 11–21).

In the study conducted by Clark et al. (2013, pp. 513–519), the researchers examined the facial areas observed by a group of 20 subjects with schizophrenia and a control group of 20 non-schizophrenic participants. The images presented to the study participants depicted emotionally neutral or angry faces (Fig. 3.1). The researchers found that:

> Schizophrenia patients required more facial information than controls to accurately differentiate between angry and neutral facial expressions, and they relied on different facial features and spatial frequencies to differentiate these facial expressions. Specifically, schizophrenia patients underutilized the eye regions, overutilized the nose and mouth regions, and virtually ignored information presented at the lowest level of spatial frequency. (Clark et al., 2013, p. 513).

---

[1] Butler et al. (2009, pp. 1095–1107), Feinberg et al. (1986, pp. 276–279), Gruzelier et al. (1999, pp. 349–362), Hooker and Park (2002, pp. 41–50), Itier and Batty (2009, pp. 843–863), Penn and Combs (2000, pp. 217–229), Whittaker et al. (2001, pp. 499–507).

[2] Addington and Addington (1998, pp. 171–181), Gold et al. (2012, pp. 424–432), Green et al. (2003, pp. 271–285), Heimberg et al. (1992, pp. 253–265), Kohler et al. (2000, pp. 127–136), Penn et al. (2002, pp. 149–159), Schneider et al. (1995, pp. 67–75), Sergi et al. (2006, pp. 448–454), Silver and Shlomo (2001, pp. 265–273), Silver et al. (2004, pp. 147–154), Silver et al. (2005, pp. 300–308), Streit et al. (1997, pp. 311–317).

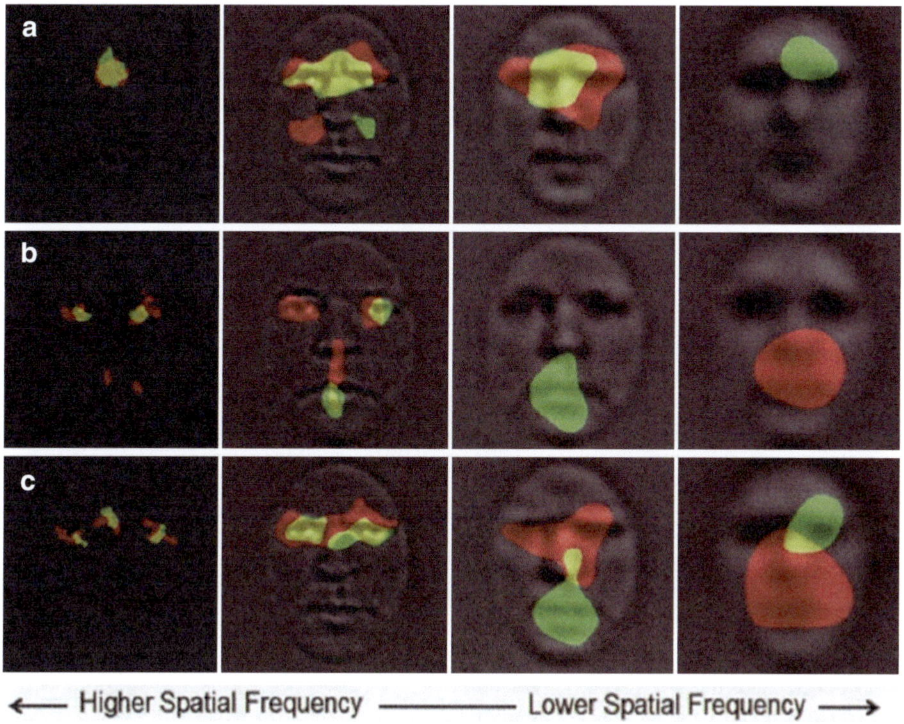

Fig. 3.1 Visual scanning of the face. The rows (**a**) and (**b**) show areas of the face significantly used by controls (red), schizophrenia patients (green), and both (yellow) in identifying angry (**a**) and neutral (**b**) expressions. Row (**c**) combines the results from above (i.e., it does not distinguish emotions) in order to show areas of the face used significantly by controls (red), schizophrenia patients (green), and by both (yellow) in distinguishing between angry and neutral faces (Clark et al., 2013, p. 516)

The result of another study conducted by a research group at the University of Lille in France is also important in this context: 20 patients with schizophrenia and 20 non-schizophrenic persons were asked to look at 40 color photos of human faces (without ears, hair, neck). Five photos presented faces known to the French public (selected from well-known artists, TV presenters, and politicians) and ten photographs presented unknown people of different ages. The remaining photos presented neutral faces of unknown adults. Pupil movements were recorded with an eye tracker.

The participants were required to identify the following:

1. The facial expressions (whether neutral, happy, sad, fearful, or angry)
2. The gender (male or female)
3. The age (whether child, adolescent, adult, or elderly)
4. Any facial familiarity (whether known or unknown)

The results of this study have given us greater insight into the gaze behavior of persons with schizophrenia. When individuals with schizophrenia look at a face passively, they do not scan all the features of the face. However, when they observe a face actively (e.g., when they have to perform a given task and are looking for something specific), their scanning of the face equals that of non-schizophrenic subjects (Nguyen et al., 2009, pp. 355–360; Yarbus, 1967) (Fig. 3.2). On the basis of these findings, it can be concluded that when guided by a precise task, even patients with schizophrenia are capable of analyzing facial expressions by observing the most important areas of a face. The researchers concluded that:

> Patients with schizophrenia exhibited reduced attention to salient facial features in the passive viewing but did not differ from controls in each active viewing (to determine the gender, the age, the emotion or the familiarity). [...] Patients in our experiments did not exhibit reduced attention to facial features in the facial expression recognition task. [...] In our study, patients fixated salient feature areas and displayed characteristically triangular scan path patterns, for all affects presented, like controls. A possible explanation is that, in the present study, participants were asked to make more active decisions (recognition of facial expression, gender, age, and assessment of familiarity) on the faces than in previous studies. This might have led participants to attend to facial features more than in the previous studies, in which participants were only asked to determine the facial expression (or view the faces passively). (Delerue et al., 2010, p. 247)

A study with children with an autism spectrum disorder has shown similar results. Although they looked into each other's eyes in a passive manner, they actively observed the others' eyes only when explicitly requested to do so (Ristic et al., 2005, pp. 715–718).

Another question is whether individuals with schizophrenia need more time to interpret a face or whether they have other deficits that qualitatively distinguish them from non-schizophrenic subjects.

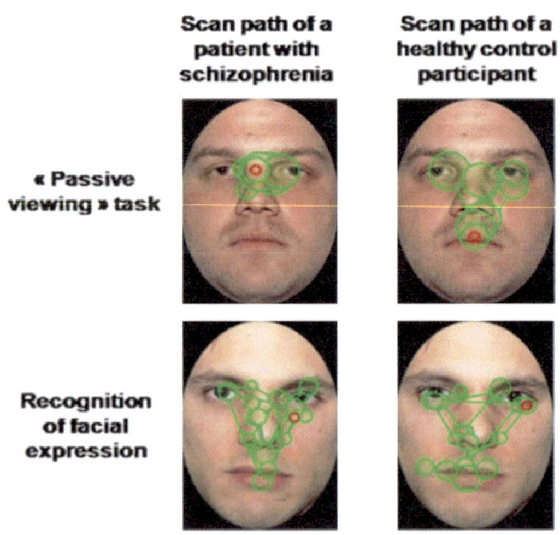

Fig. 3.2 Eye tracking test in passive and active vision (Delerue et al., 2010, p. 247)

To measure the reaction time in face recognition, an experiment was conducted with 20 male subjects with chronic schizophrenia and 16 non-schizophrenic male subjects between the ages of 20 and 55 (Onitsuka et al., 2006, pp. 455–462).

The aim of the experiment was to examine whether individuals with schizophrenia show a lower activation of the neuronal networks when looking at a human face than the non-schizophrenic subjects in the control group. In addition, both groups were required to perform another task involving the recognition of a frequently used object such as a car.

The stimuli, to which the study participants were exposed, were 32 color photographs of emotionally neutral faces. Of the 32 presented faces, 16 were male, 16 female, 16 Asian, and 16 Caucasian. Previous studies using EEG have revealed that non-schizophrenic subjects show an N170 potential which is specifically related to seeing faces but not to other objects. Therefore, the N170 wave can be used as a physiological index that indicates facial recognition (Bentin et al., 1996, pp. 551–565; Watanabe et al., 1999, pp. 125–142). Onitsuka and his colleagues state:

> We found that schizophrenia patients, relative to non-schizophrenic comparison subjects, showed bilateral N170 amplitude reduction specifically in response to images of faces (it is important to note that no stimulus effect was observed in the patients group). (Onitsuka et al., 2006, p. 460)

There is no difference in the response to the auto-stimulus between non-schizophrenic subjects and subjects with schizophrenia, but there is a significant difference in the response to the face stimulus between the two groups. Thus, the findings of the study are strongly suggestive that there exists a face recognition impairment in individuals with schizophrenia.

This impairment of the ability to interpret faces and emotions can be explained as follows: A frame enables one to understand what is represented within the frame as a whole. Even with regard to the human face, individuals with schizophrenia do not seem to be able to frame the various elements of the face into a unified *Gestalt* (in the sense of *Gestalt psychology*). This is evidenced by the observation that these individuals tend not to observe the face as a whole, but only parts of it spontaneously. Clark, Gosselin, and Goghari are emphatic on this idea:

> Schizophrenia patients demonstrate a restricted scanning strategy involving shorter scan path lengths, fewer fixations, increased fixation duration, and notable avoidance of relevant facial features irrespective of emotional valence. Consistent with deficits in early-stage low spatial frequency integration, results from this area have suggested that patients have difficulties in conceptualizing an "initial face" predisposing them to fragmented sequential processing of all features of the face, rather than gestalt perception of the face and its particularly salient emotional features. (Clark et al., 2013, p. 518)

The metaphor of the frame also has its explanatory power here: The inability to recognize emotional expressions in other faces impairs the perception of the feelings and the perspective of those with whom we interact.

3.3 Body Language

The first milestone in the research on body language in modern times is Charles Darwin's famous work *The Expression of the Emotions in Man and Animals* (1872/1999). During the twentieth century, many scientists studied non-verbal communication and body language. Among these are Paul Ekman, who has devoted many studies to understanding facial expressions (Ekman & Scherer, 1982; Ekman, 2016; Bateson, 1972, pp. 218–235, 413–428), and Ray Birdwhistell, who was inspired by descriptive linguistics, and went on to create a grammar of body language that was analogous to the grammar of a spoken language (Birdwhistell, 1970). Alexander Lowen noted that bodily attitudes can be traced back to the person's emotional or existential attitudes (Lowen, 1958). The physiology of body language was the sine qua non for studying the deficits present in some neurological and psychiatric pathologies.

While there have not yet been many studies on the perception of body language in individuals with schizophrenia, particular patterns have already become apparent.

Thoma et al. (2013, pp. 1152–1163) used EEG to investigate the neurological responses of P100 and N170 in two groups of subjects which included 14 patients with schizophrenia treated in the psychiatric department of the Ruhr University Bochum and 15 non-schizophrenic individuals, all aged between 20 and 53 years. The EEG analyses showed a correlation between visual stimulation (facial and body expression) and the evoked potentials P100 and N170. Nonprofessional actors simulated sadness, fear, joy, or a neutral facial expression together with the corresponding body postures (Fig. 3.3). The actors were masked so that respondents were not distracted by stimuli from the actors' faces. To avoid further distraction, the actors also wore trousers, preferably dark ones, and black t-shirts. The study participants were requested to answer questions about the perceived identity of the persons (the actors) and the emotional value of the proxemics. The persons could be the same or

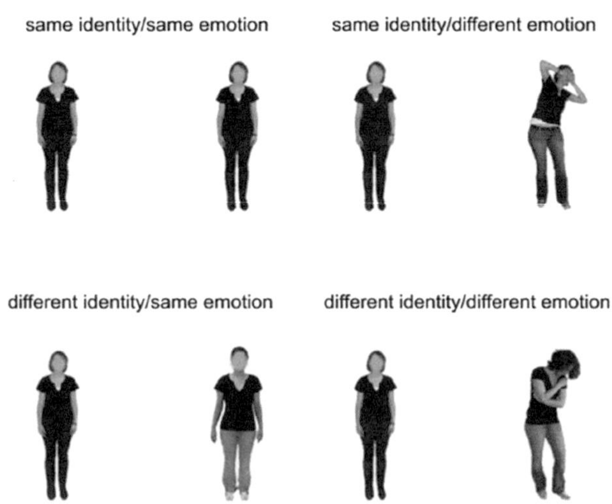

Fig. 3.3 Body language and interpretation of emotions (Thoma et al., 2013, p. 1155)

different each time (identity question) and take different emotional postures (emotion question).

The experiment (Fig. 3.4) is conducted as follows: At the beginning, a dot on a display is shown for between 100 and 400 ms. Then, an image (face or body) appears for 1 s. This is followed by a neutral screen for 200 ms and a white screen for 400 ms. Finally, the last image (face or body) is displayed together with a visual stimulus for 2 s.

The following graphs show the response of patients with schizophrenia and non-schizophrenic subjects as well as the difference in the amplitude of their responses in the EEG (Figs. 3.6 and 3.7; here, SZ is the label for a schizophrenia patient and HC for a member of the healthy control group).

P7 and P8 are 2 of the 30 electrodes used in the EEG protocol:

> Inspection of the grand mean waveforms showed that maximal or minimal amplitudes were seen at electrode positions P7 and P8. The statistical analysis focused on the P100 and N170. P100 and N170 maxima were determined as peak amplitudes between 80 and 130 ms (P100) and 130 and 210 ms (N170). Amplitude maxima were used to determine P100 and N170 latencies. (Thoma et al., 2013, p. 1156)

By comparing the graphs of the two groups (Figs. 3.5 and 3.6), we can conclude that there is a notable difference in response between the SZ and the HC participants.

> The aim of the current study was to investigate whether impaired processing of emotional faces in schizophrenia is paralleled by processing of emotions expressed by human bodies, both on the behavioral level and in terms of ERPs. We also aimed to elucidate whether these potential alterations are affected by emotional or personal identity of the face/bodies. To summarize the most relevant findings involving the group factor, patients with schizophrenia showed overall poorer behavioral performance (fewer correct responses and longer response times) than non-schizophrenic controls, irrespective of stimulus category (bodies vs. faces) and personal or emotional identity (same vs. different). Relating response times to the proportion of correct responses using inverse efficiency scores in order to control for speed-accuracy trade-offs revealed overall lower response efficiency in the patients relative to controls, across all conditions. Patients also showed overall more misses than controls, particularly for bodies. (Thoma et al., 2013, p. 1159)

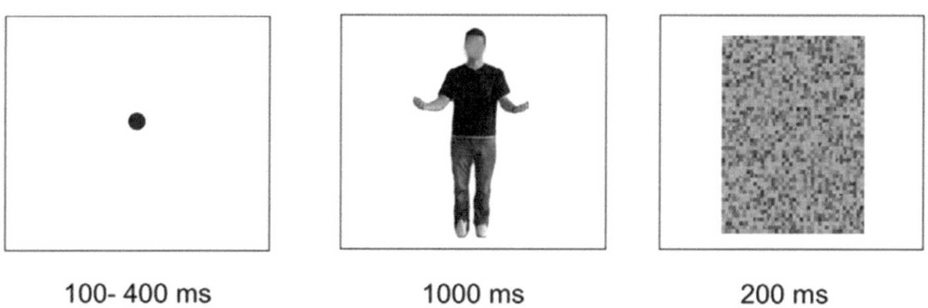

Fig. 3.4 Thomas's experiment (Thoma et al., 2013, p. 1155)

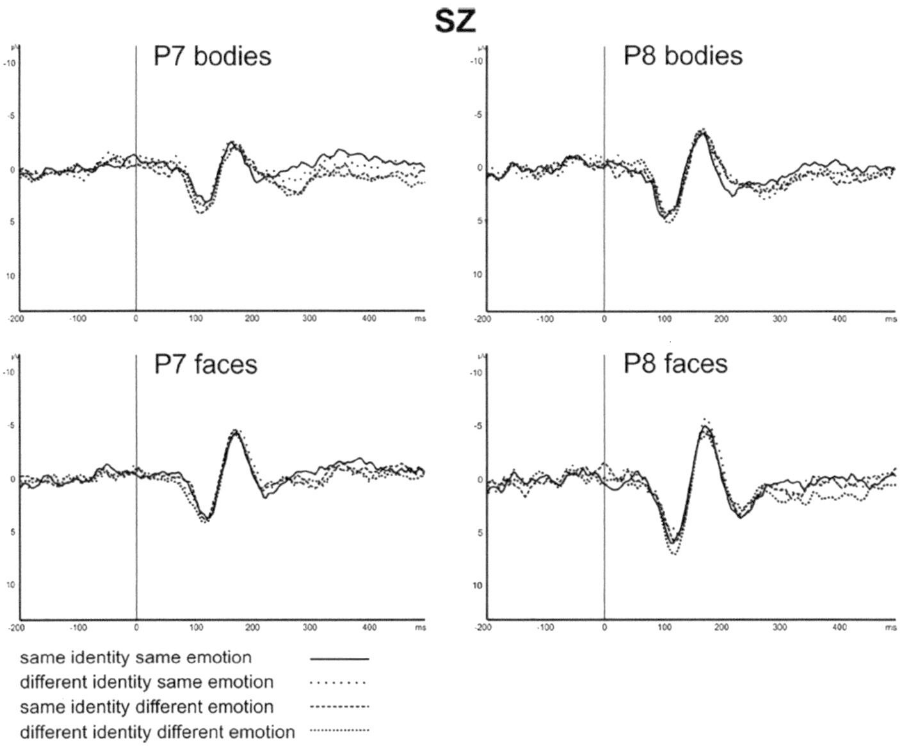

Fig. 3.5 EEG amplitudes of patients with schizophrenia in Thomas's experiment (Thoma et al., 2013, p. 1158)

A further study conducted by Vaskinn et al. (2016, pp. 1–7) aimed at analyzing the reactions of individuals with schizophrenia and non-schizophrenic subjects to several emotional stimuli of body language: anger, happiness, sadness, fear, and an emotionally neutral posture (Fig. 3.7). The experiment included 60 individuals with schizophrenia, 24 with schizoaffective disorder, and 185 non-schizophrenic (healthy) persons. All of the study participants were in a clinically stable state. As a result, compared to non-schizophrenic subjects, patients with schizophrenia showed impairment in their perception of emotions. Frequently, both happiness and neutral emotional states were often perceived more accurately than anger and particularly fear.

The consistent deficit in reading body language in the group of the patients with schizophrenia seems to point to a general problem.

Other studies have been conducted in the neuropsychiatric field to investigate the links between the phenomenology of understanding emotions and neurobiological changes in schizophrenic individuals (Viher et al., 2017, pp. 213–221).

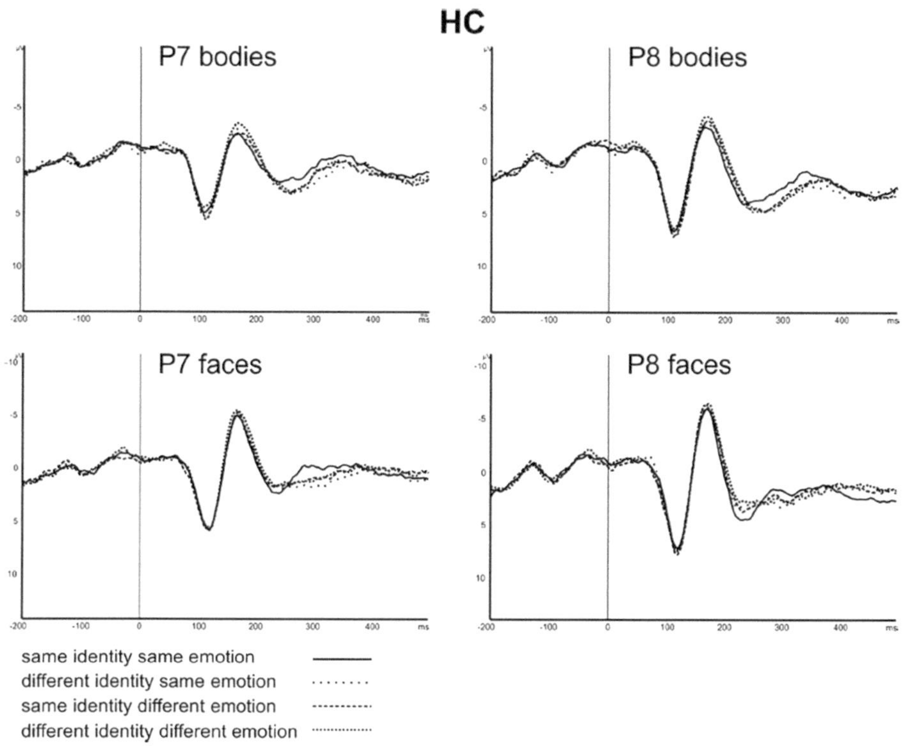

Fig. 3.6 EEG amplitudes of non-schizophrenic (healthy) subjects in Thomas's experiment (Thoma et al., 2013, p. 1159)

Fig. 3.7 Comparison between non-schizophrenic (healthy) subjects (HC) and patients with schizophrenia (SZ) in the body language reading test (Vaskinn et al., 2016, p. 5)

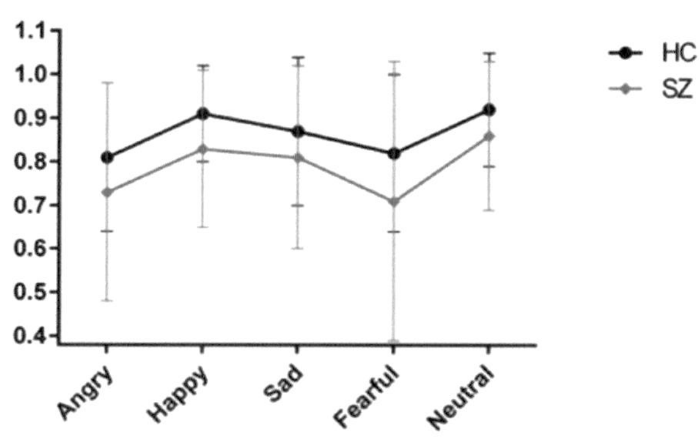

Studies on body language conducted with patients with schizophrenia reveal that individuals with schizophrenia show clear deficits in understanding other people's emotions manifesting in proxemics and body gestures. Failing to comprehend body language suggests a corresponding failure to understand the emotional perspective of other people and the emotional reactions that one triggers in them. As with any spoken language, body language provides a means of communication that ensures mutual understanding, however, only as long as you can "read" body language. When two or more people speak different languages or with different emotional interpretations (as is the case with schizophrenia), the risk of mutual misunderstanding is very high, and the interlocutors construct independent frames. Body language creates a shared and coded framework within which certain gestures, postures, and attitudes should be mutually correctly interpreted in order for communication not to result in a failure and misunderstanding.

3.4 Summary

Perceiving and comprehending the emotions of others quickly and with clarity is a prerequisite for a healthy social life. Recently, many studies have found serious deficits in patients with schizophrenia in both facial and emotion perception and in correctly comprehending body language. Incomplete exploration of other people's faces is the reason for the difficulties individuals with schizophrenia have in adequately understanding emotions. The impaired ability to interpret faces, emotions, and body language is represented in the *frame theory* as follows: A frame enables one to understand what is represented in it as a whole. Even in relation to the human face or body, individuals with schizophrenia seem to be unable to frame the various elements of the face or body into a unified *Gestalt* (in the sense of *Gestalt psychology*). This results in an impaired intersubjective understanding of emotional and nonverbal communication.

Analysis of Artistic Expressions 4

4.1 Introduction

This chapter describes artistic expressions of individuals with schizophrenia within the *subjectivity-frame-perspective theory*. The main thesis here is that impairments similar to the language disorders or difficulties in understanding nonverbal language observed in individuals with schizophrenia can also be found in their perspectival and unified representation of artistic expressions. A perspectival and unified representation is guaranteed and conceived by the frame. Lack of perspective and frame, which are evident in artistic expressions and artworks of individuals with schizophrenia, is to be correlated with the impairment of the subjectivity of the representing subject or with its ontological instability.

4.2 Art and Schizophrenia

The artistic expressions of individuals with schizophrenia are fascinating and have attracted the attention of many scholars, physicians, art critics, and philosophers for decades. It has often been debated whether drawings, paintings, sculptures, or other artefacts created by individuals with schizophrenia should be considered as art or not. In this book, the artistic expressions of individuals with schizophrenia are regarded as signs of their ability to perceive and create. In this chapter, the term *art* is thus used in a broader sense than in art history and art criticism and includes all figurative representations of patients with schizophrenia. The artistic production of individuals with schizophrenia is thus considered from a clinical-phenomenological perspective. The artwork of schizophrenia patients, as with all art, is individual expression of perceptions and, as such, can be analyzed and interpreted to yield data on how individuals with schizophrenia (in comparison with control groups) perceive and depict the world.

P. Parisi, *A Phenomenological Interpretation of Schizophrenia*,
https://doi.org/10.1007/978-3-031-67860-8_4

The hypothesis here is that works of art created by individuals with schizophrenia show parallels to their linguistic expressions and to their way of perceiving space and time: Figurative representations by individuals with schizophrenia are often characterized by a fragmentary style and the absence of a coherent overall structure, a naturalistic three-dimensional spatiality, as well as a comprehensible conceptual and spatial relationship between the depicted elements. Frequently, also an obsessive repetition of a graphic element or a rigidity of a two-dimensional geometrism can be observed.

What is important about this hypothesis is that *looseness* of association manifests itself clearly not only at the linguistic level but also at the level of artistic representation. The looseness of syntax and other linguistic disorders typical of linguistic expressions produced by individual with schizophrenia corresponds, in art, to the absence of a figurative syntax capable of imparting order to the various parts of a whole. In this sense, from a conceptual point of view, the role and meaning of the frame seems to be ignored in schizophrenic art. The frame creates that a priori space in which the various objects can be placed: The frame is the expression of a subject who knows it and can see through it, in a perspectival way. The artistic expressions of individuals with schizophrenia show, as Blankenburg points out, the "loss of natural self-evidence" (Blankenburg, 1991).

Prior to analyzing the impairment of frame (frame as a guarantor of the general unity of the artwork) and perspective (as an element of affirmation of the subject in the world of naturalistic representation), the question whether and how schizophrenic disorder and artistic style correlate needs to be examined. Such a correlation can be shown in biographically contextualizable artworks.

In the following three clinical and artistic examples, we will explore how schizophrenic symptomatology and its remission are reflected through a change of style within the artistic work collection of a schizophrenia patient.

4.2.1 Louis Wain

The first artist who will be discussed both chronologically and because of his paradigmatic importance in the literature is Louis Wain (Dale, 1968; Damiani & Fusar-Poli, 2018, p. 315; McGennis, 1999, p. 27 f.). Born in London in 1860, he was unable to attend school until he was 10 years old owing to his physical weakness. After attending the *West London School of Art,* he commenced employment as a teacher and illustrator. At 24 years of age, he married Emily Richardson. However, soon after this, she was diagnosed with breast cancer. To comfort himself over his wife's pain, Louis Wain brought home a black and white cat whom thy named Peter. Although he had never painted cats before, Peter became his favorite subject of his artwork and in time Wain established himself as a cat illustrator. In 1886, the newspaper *Illustrated London News commissioned him to* make a drawing known as *A Kitten's Christmas Party,* which was perhaps the peak of Louis Wain's fame. The death of the artist's sister and his beloved cat contributed to the artist's mental exhaustion. He became increasingly paranoid and fell into a morbid psychosis.

After physically assaulting his sisters, he was eventually isolated in a psychiatric ward, where he remained until his death in 1939. Although it is difficult to precisely correlate the artist's change in style with the progression of his mental disorder, the developing mental illness is mirrored by a change in his artistic style of depiction (Fig. 4.1).

The four paintings, which are part of a huge *corpus* of illustrations, attest the process of artistic transformation: from the naturalistic representation of a cat's head in its three-dimensionality and in the roundness of its forms and volumes to a representation that is completely flat, two-dimensional, and characterized by an absolute geometry and symmetry. Even though this last representation is well placed in the center of the sheet, it possesses neither a special perspective nor reference to the frame. The frame is missing because the drawing does not stand a priori in the space. The geometry of the figure follows rules of extension and development internal to the drawing. The two-dimensional space of the geometry in paintings created by individuals with schizophrenia is a space that evolves together with the figure and not before. There is no a priori space in which the figures are situated. The space is not an a priori three-dimensional space but instead a two-dimensional space and representation while the frame is part of the unthought in Wain's later work. The fourth picture of the cat (Fig. 4.1d) represents one of the possible developments of schizophrenic art, namely, a development towards geometrism. It would thus appear that the mental disorder prompted substantial changes in the artistic style of the cat illustrations.

4.2.2 Pfeifer's Patient

The second example showing that schizophrenic disorders are manifest in a change in an artist's representational abilities is provided by Richard Arwed Pfeifer's book on schizophrenic art *Der Geisteskranke und sein Werk. Eine Studie über schizophrene Kunst* (Literally: The mentally ill and his work. A study on schizophrenic art) from 1923.

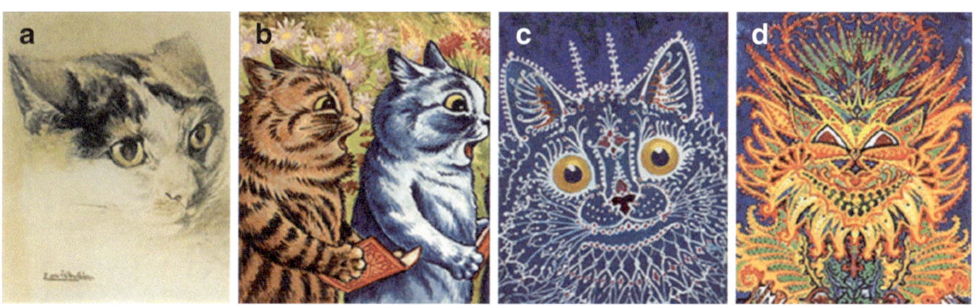

Fig. 4.1 (**a**–**d**) Louis Wain's change of style during the development of his schizophrenia (Damiani & Fusar-Poli, 2018, p. 315)

As in the case of Louis Wain, Pfeifer's patient is a skilled illustrator (Fig. 4.2a) who, at some point in her life, possibly also triggered by the immense emotional pain due to the premature loss of her young husband, developed a schizophrenia disorder. In his book, Richard Arwed Pfeifer provides a detailed portrait of the young woman's childhood, education, and bereavement. He emphasizes that she "developed quite normally," that she was considered clever, "half a child prodigy." She attended an industrial school and then an art academy, where she assimilated and complied with the acceptable academic styles as a very good student with "strict school discipline." At the age of 21, she married a landscape painter she had met at the academy. Pfeifer reports how this promising life collapsed only 5 months after her marriage:

> Her husband (went) to the field and did not return. In St. Quentin, she was able to stay with him for 14 days. After his amputation, he died of gas phlegmon. The relatives thought that the horror of what she had seen and experienced must have been too much for her. She seemed to have forgotten even how to cry. She bore her fate with heroic coldness, never complained, never told of the last time she and her husband were together, never cried. [...] In the meantime she was working as a craftswoman. (Pfeifer, 1923, p. 75 f.; source in German).

Pfeifer then describes the woman's psychological suffering, her feeling of emptiness, and her snake hallucinations (Fig. 4.2b shows a snake in the Snow Queen's basket).

The artistic style of this patient shows profound transformations: Fig. 4.2c shows a woman in profile, just two-dimensional, without a background. Above her head,

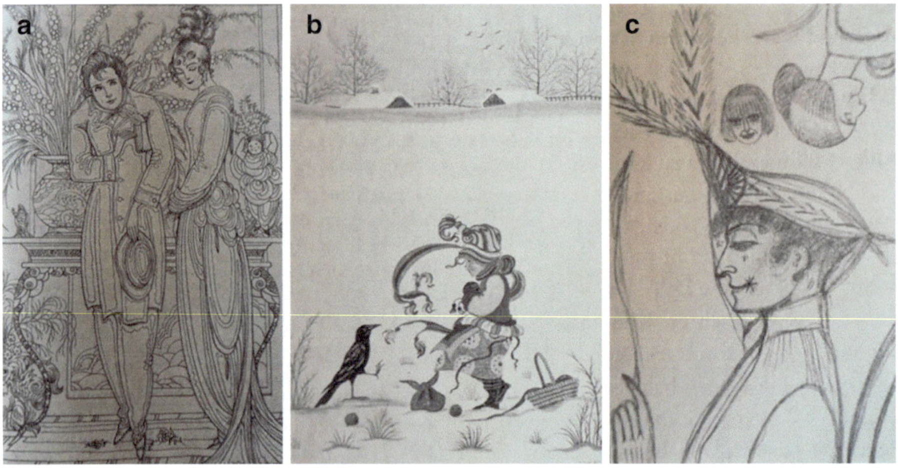

Fig. 4.2 (**a–c**) Drawings by Pfeifer's patient. (**a**) Illustration sample from the novel; the woman's costume contains clear reminiscences of mannequins. The contours of the man's suit are emphasized in a mannered way. (**b**) 'Snow Queen'. A snake not supposed to be in the fairy tale crawls into the basket (hallucination). (**c**) Drawing of the artist after 2 years of illness" (Pfeifer, 1923, pp. 77, 80, 83)

there are two other heads that appear isolated and in strange positions. The loss of cohesion and coherence is a feature typical of paintings and drawings by artists with schizophrenia. Pfeifer notes that the third drawing (Fig. 4.2c) was made by the patient 2 years after the onset of schizophrenia.

4.2.3 Little Franz

The third example linking schizophrenia with a change of artistic style is from the famous work *Schizophrenia and Art* by Navratil (1965). The name of Navratil's patient was Franz. His psychiatric treatment started at the age of 17. Franz was born deaf and at the age of 17 looked like a 13-year-old child. He could only articulate a few sounds and a few words, could only count to five, and was innumerate. Franz communicated chiefly by means of drawings. In the first years of his stay in the psychiatric hospital, he showed severe behavioral disorders that fluctuated between outbursts of rage and need for love. He enjoyed reproducing illustrations with pencil, and he was skilled in that (Fig. 4.3).

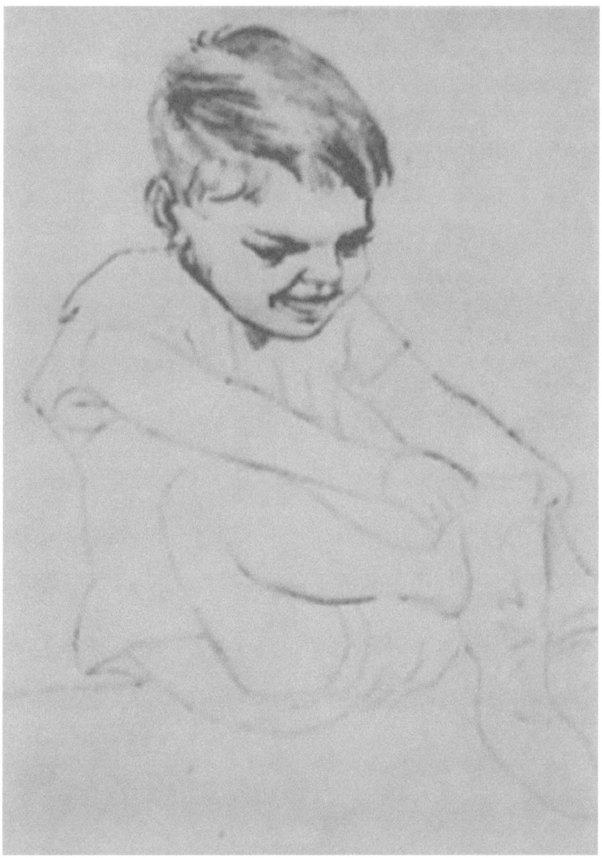

Fig. 4.3 Franz: before the onset of psychosis (Navratil, 1965, p. 43)

At the age of 24, the first signs of psychosis became apparent. This phase of his schizophrenia was characterized by insomnia, immobility during the day, and indifference to his surroundings. Then, he spent a few months in bed in an autistic-like state, hiding his head under the covers. He was no longer able, as Navratil reports, to make the simplest mosaics by means of cubes. This clinical picture not only illustrates Franz's attitude of rejection but is also important for diagnosing a deficit in the ability to handle an overall picture.

During the psychosis, Franz was no longer master of his drawings. The following picture (Fig. 4.4) was created during his psychotic phase before the treatment.

Franz underwent electroshock therapy, which improved his health. He began to draw again and showed renewed interest and pleasure in this beloved activity of his. However, the psychosis and the treatment had left their mark on the young man's mind, and his drawings were no longer what they once were. Navratil describes the change in style and perspective as follows:

> [The picture] is covered with figures and scribbles right up to the edge. One recognizes buildings in distorted perspective, animals, a single eye, and spiral-like lines. The continuous vertical orientation of the drawing sheet, which was rotated by the invalid while drawing, is missing. (Navratil, 1965, p. 45; source in German)

In the course of the treatment, Franz's pictures continued to display a distorted representation of space and a loss of inner coherence: They showed figures of different kinds heaped on top of each other in a chaotic way and without any general compositional frame of reference (Figs. 4.5 and 4.6).

> As the treatment progressed, the psychotic symptoms became more pronounced again. The buildings that Franz was drawing now show an accelerated perspective and appear to fall off

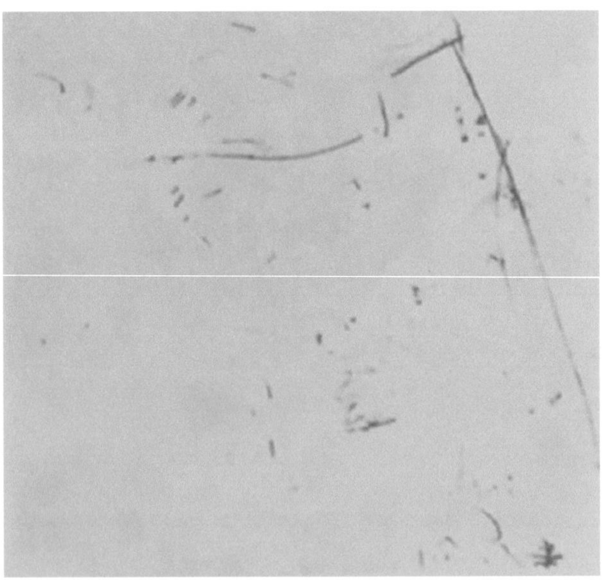

Fig. 4.4 A drawing by Franz at the peak of psychosis (Navratil, 1965, p. 44)

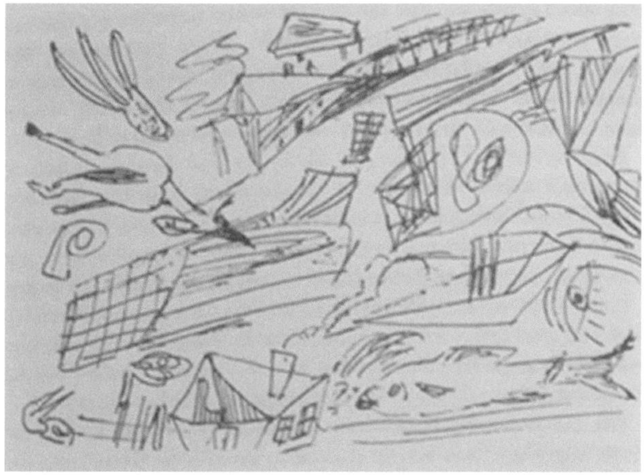

Fig. 4.5 A drawing by Franz during the course of treatment (I) (Navratil, 1965, p. 46)

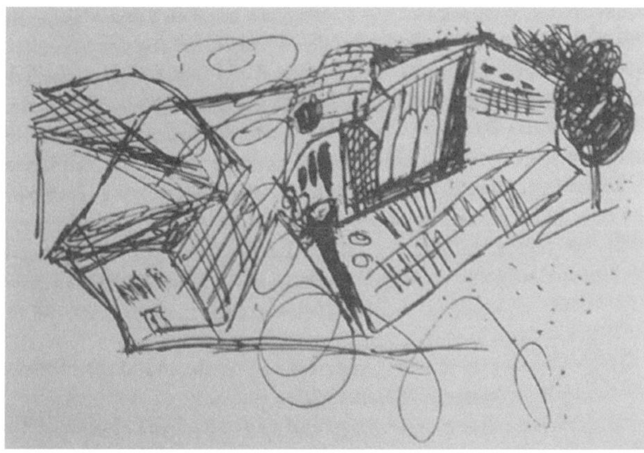

Fig. 4.6 A drawing by Franz during the course of treatment (II) (Navratil, 1965, p. 46)

> the space. The spiral-shaped line in the center of the picture reinforces the impression of being in a whirl. [...]. After the end of the convulsive treatment (with a total of 12 convulsions), the patient could no longer produce a drawing with a higher structure. (Navratil, 1965, p. 45, p. 47; source in German)

Franz's drawings lack a consistent form during this phase. On the contrary, during the second psychotic relapse, the young patient returns to childish scribbling (Figs. 4.7 and 4.8).

> A second electroconvulsive treatment was started 63 days after completion of the first convulsive series. The mental state of the patient was as bad as before the first treatment. Only 2 h after the triggering of a new seizure, the patient was able to draw a human form again. (Navratil, 1965, p. 50; source in German)

About 3 months after the start of the second treatment, Franz was in a better mental state than in the prepsychotic phase. The characteristic features of schizophrenia seem to have disappeared from his drawings completely or almost

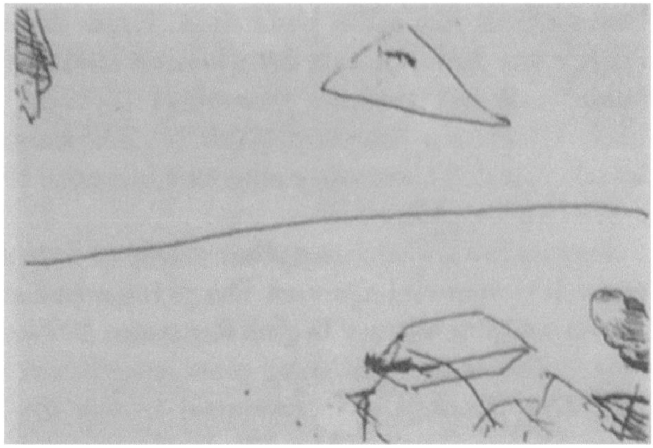

Fig. 4.7 A drawing by Franz during psychotic relapse (I) (Navratil, 1965, p. 49)

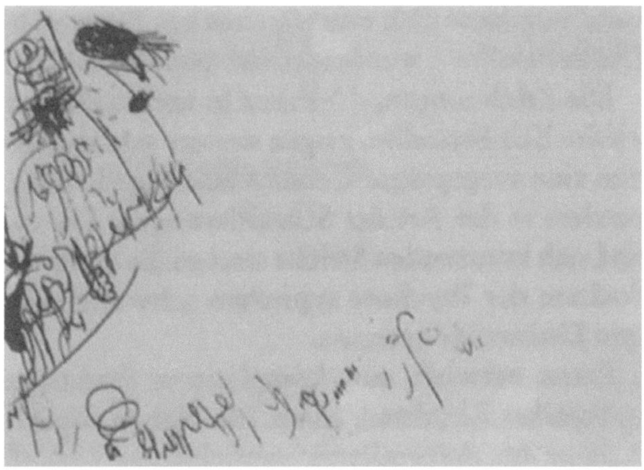

Fig. 4.8 A drawing by Franz during psychotic relapse (II) (Navratil, 1965, p. 49)

completely. Franz's ability to draw portraits has returned, as the illustrations in Figs. 4.9, 4.10, and 4.11 show. Franz's radically improved graphic production clearly reflects the improvement in his mental abilities.

In the following words, Leo Navratil provides a general analysis of the artistic biography of the young Franz, which is to be read in the context of the outstanding events in the history of the patient's illness:

> Rarely does one have the opportunity to observe the drawing of a person who is so gifted in drawing and so largely isolated from environmental influences before the onset of a schizophrenic psychosis, at its peak, during the course of treatment and healing, and after the onset of full remission. On the basis of the material we have collected, consisting of more than 300 individual drawings, we can state the following: The drawings of our patient lacked any relationship to the real outside world during his mental disorder, but they conveyed deep insights into his inner world. The healing is indicated by a gradual but finally full attention to the things and people of his environment. Thus, the depictive function of

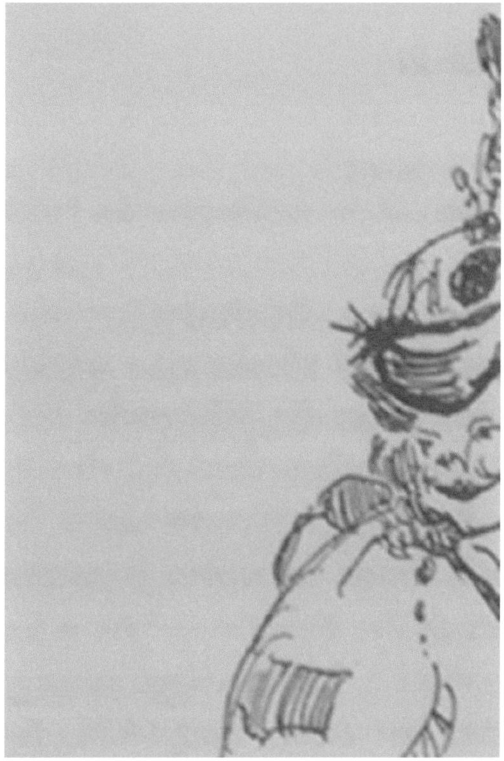

Fig. 4.9 A drawing by Franz after renewed treatment (Navratil, 1965, p. 51)

drawing, which had been missing during the mental illnesses, came to the fore again. The change in style that radically took place in this case consists of a transition from lifelike to anti-naturalistic representation and a return to naturalism after the psychosis had subsided. Finally, the drawings created by our patient during the psychosis show numerous Mannerist features: Enigmatic symbolic images, eerie and grotesque or floating figures, a peculiar contrast of motion and rigidity, deformation phenomena and constructivist tendencies, accelerated perspective and spinning space, the maze-like intertwined line, picture puzzle-like drawings, the single eye and the motifs of death, the mirror, the mask. (Navratil, 1965, pp. 53–55; source in German).

The examples of the artists presented above reveal a close connection between schizophrenia and features in the figurative art created by individuals with schizophrenia. Just as the disorders of schizophrenic thinking manifest themselves as disorders of language, they also become apparent in changes in figurative drawing and painting. Therefore, in the artworks created by individuals with schizophrenia, one can find close phenomenological equivalents in the fragmentary and restructured manner of perceiving space, in the perspective, in the general coherence, and in the unified vision of the whole in these patients.

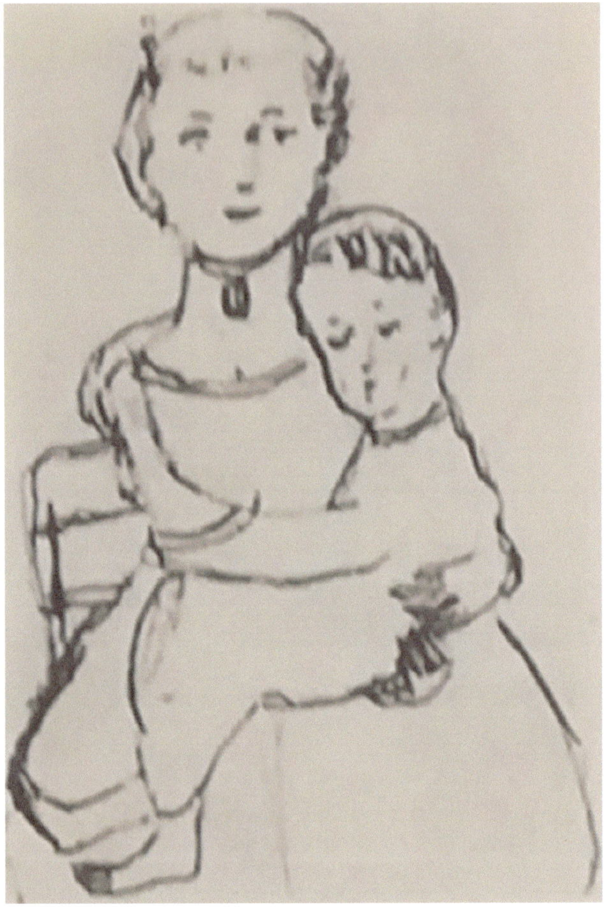

Fig. 4.10 A drawing by Franz after healing (I) (Navratil, 1965, p. 54)

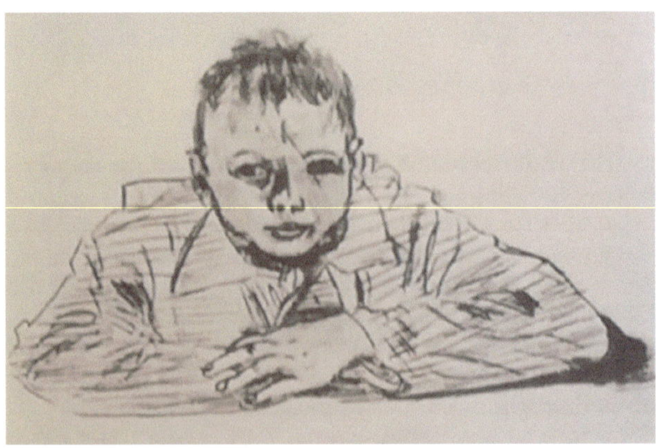

Fig. 4.11 A drawing by Franz after healing (II) (Navratil, 1965, p. 54)

4.3 Frame

A frame is that element which makes it possible to distinguish the inner from the outer, the adequate from the inadequate. The frame guarantees a unified picture and gives the work coherence in form and content.

When panel painting (both as an object and also as an art form) and frame (in its Renaissance version) were born at the beginning of the early modern period (fifteenth century), a certain theory of vision emerged: The theory of perspective, according to which all represented objects are uniformly aligned to a vanishing point. The vanishing point defines the perspective of a subject from whose point of view all represented objects are arranged. Perspective developed from a transcendental concept of the subject. It is no coincidence that other cultures, which did not develop this transcendental concept of the subject to such an extent, also did not conceive of a theory of perspective.

Attention to perspectival composition is classically present not only in the visual arts but also in literature (especially in the literary genre of poetry), music, architecture, and other artistical fields. In our time, we do not recognize absolute values of these forms and proportions anymore, because the main currents of art today are characterized by their radical deconstruction of the old concepts of beauty and harmony (Boehm, 2007, pp. 229–242; Sass, 1992). The principles of classical composition harmonize the particular and the general, which become part of a regulated order of proportions and spatiality. What aesthetics traditionally called *beauty* was the harmony of parts, which is based on the principle of proportionality.

The works of figurative art created by individuals with schizophrenia, whether it is drawings or paintings, appear to suspend the principles of unified composition. The elements in the drawings appear in a random, chaotic, disordered, or serial order of association; the drawings seem to be *expandable* at will. Therefore, the concept of frame finds no place in schizophrenic art.

The problem of the frame (and thus of cohesion and coherence) is addressed in the scientific literature by, for instance, Navratil (1965), Rennert (1962), and Röske (1995). There is certainly no fixed set of features characteristic of all artworks created by artists with schizophrenia. As with any human phenomenon, there exists an individual, cultural, biographical variability. In the following, we will consider the effects of schizophrenia patients' inability to pursue a coherent thought, even when this thought appears to dominate the scene (as is the case with geometrism or the orderly repetition of individual objects), on the appearance of their artistic objects.

An example of incoherence in works by individuals with schizophrenia is an example of thematic incoherence. Heterogeneous elements are presented in one and the same drawing not for reasons of overall coherence but for pure juxtaposition. The frame plays no role in the overall organization of the content.

The drawings which will be discussed here are constructed as follows: In the first drawing, a large horse in the center of the sheet is surrounded by smaller, repetitive elements. The horse has a small torso and long strong legs, and its head is drooping. It appears detached, not subject to gravity. It floats freely in an ethereal space, which also applies to the many small repetitive figures of women and flowers.

In the second drawing, the overall structure is similar: A large musical instrument occupies the center of the sheet and is surrounded by female figures with muscular bodies. The women in the first and second drawing are similar and appear naked and in clearly erotic positions. In the drawing with the musical instrument, an erotic scene in which a man penetrates a woman can be observed on the right side.

In both works, there is a formal and thematic heterogeneity of the central figure and the surrounding figures.

However, there is an inconsistency in the depiction of the main objects in the works. The horse is depicted with a drooping head, in a sad or meditative or tired posture. There is also a clear inconsistency in the elements that distinguish the work: The title of the work informs us that it is a horse; however, it has a mottled skin like a cow and the ears and physical features of a donkey. These are among the inconsistencies of the painting. A further inconsistency can be noted in the relationship between the subject matter of the central figure and the surrounding figures.

In the second drawing, the musical instrument has some heart-shaped decorations on the edge, which are the result of the artist's free association, perhaps in reference to the female eroticism evident in the work.

A further distinctive type of pictorial representations created by artists with schizophrenia in which the frame loses its graphical and theoretical meaning can be observed in drawings in which the same object is repeated several times. The pure seriality, based on the indefinite quantitative repetition of an element, renders the frame qualitatively ineffective. These works have in common that they present a repetition of the same object. The artist had spread the drawn figures to the physical edges of the sheet on which he is drawing. It is conceivable that the artist could have repeated the objects infinitely if the sheet would be boundless. In such forms of representation, the frame does not exist: The only limit is a physical (the sheet of paper in its materiality) and not a conceptual one. Instead of formal coherence, one can observe an obsession here: An indefinite multiplication of the same element that the artist seeks to capture again and again by drawing it because it would not leave his mind. Likewise, a representational repetition suggests an effort of the will to render the object present always and everywhere. The chairs, like the other objects, hang on the surface without depth.

Two fundamental aspects of such serial images are as follows:

1. The entire work is formed by simple repetition of a single object.
2. The frame can be extended indefinitely without changing the meaning of the work. Meanwhile, the frame loses both its differentiating and organizing function.

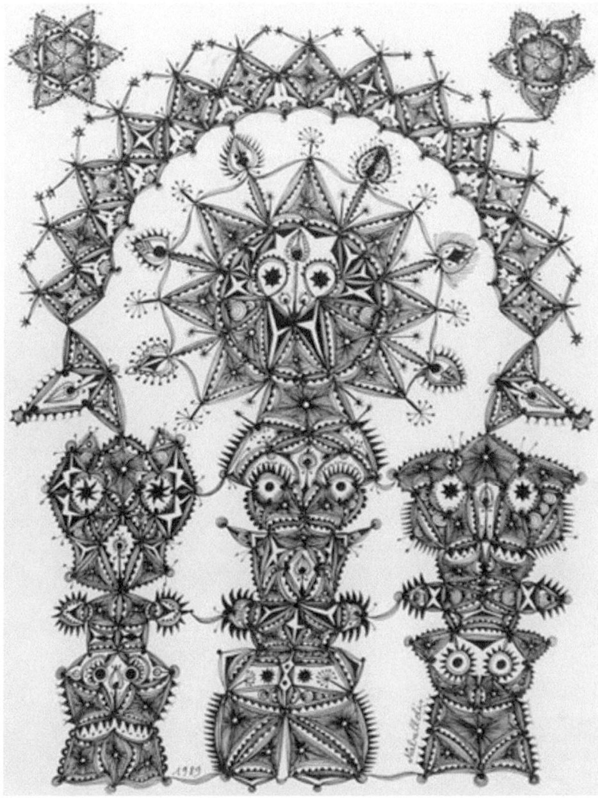

Fig. 4.12 Marc Lamy, *Naballelino, 1989* (Landert, 2011, p. 293)

Another characteristic feature which is often observed in artworks created by individuals with schizophrenia is geometrism. At first glance, geometric images, which are constructed in different symmetries, seem to be based on a holistic concept. The first example of geometrism that was discussed here is the drawings by Louis Wain, in which the cats' heads increasingly take on a simple, flattened, symmetrical, and Mannerist ornamented form.

The following drawings by Marc Lamy and Marco Raugei are examples of animal figures (resembling owls, Fig. 4.12) and plants (sunflowers, Fig. 4.13) that are not presented in an organically vital manner but instead in an ornamentally rigid manner. The geometry of the depicted elements seems to indicate an attempt to cling to a graphic certainty where everything is controlled and ordered, which is possibly an artistic compensation for a fundamental uncertainty in the way patients with schizophrenia experience themselves and their world.[1] There is no trace of emotion in these drawings, apart from the eyes, which in Marc Lamy's drawing is wide open and staring. The sunflowers are fixed in an unnatural immobility.

[1] Cf. Minkowski (1927, pp. 63–80).

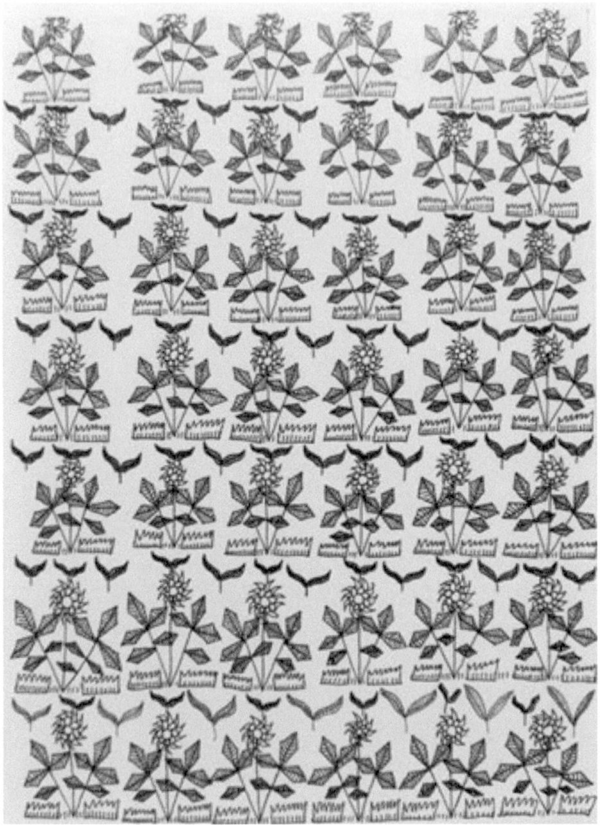

Fig. 4.13 Marco Raugei, *Sunflowers*, 1993 (Landert, 2011, p. 299)

Valerie Potter's works are a striking example of strict geometry (Fig. 4.14). In these works, the artist seems to master the general order and the general scheme very well. Her hand is certainly steadier and perhaps her mind sharper than those of many other patients with schizophrenia who draw in a clumsier or more disorganized way. The two works are made with great technical skill, but, and this is of fundamental importance, they say nothing about the artist's lifeworld or state of mind. Her subjectivity remains out of the representation. The geometrism in schizophrenia patients' artworks thus lacks perspectivity.

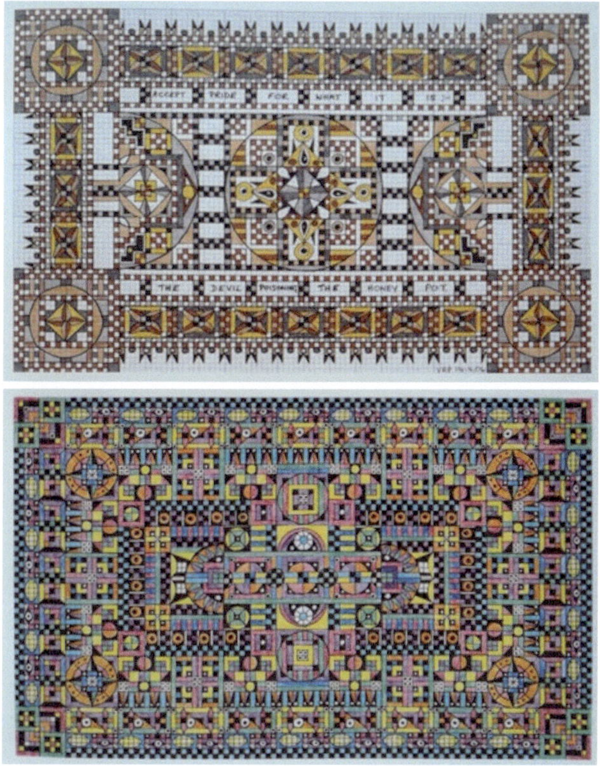

Fig. 4.14 Valerie Potter, *Accept for what it is*, 2006; *Untitled, 2007* (Landert, 2011, p. 327)

4.4 Perspective

The pictures discussed so far show another common feature: It can be observed that the perspective is uncertain, sketchy, or even completely absent. This is no coincidence. The frame problem implies the perspective problem and vice versa. This problematic rooted in the problematic of subjectivity renders an incapability of gaining an objectifying view of the world. Perspective and frame mediate between the perceiving subject and the object being perceived. The Latin word *obiectum* (in German *Objekt*) is constructed similarly to the German lexeme *Gegenstand*. *Obiectum* is originally an *ob-iectum*; *ob-* means *before* and *iectum* is the past participle of the verb *iacere*, which literally means *to throw*. The German term *Gegenstand* (object) means literally "that, which stands against."

In the objective and factual relationship, the subject must gain a certain distance that allows the subject to see and to see itself. In order to be able to recognize the other, it is necessary to presuppose an *I*.

Perspectival drawing and painting were developed from the attempt to depict spatial relationships of objects in relation to the viewer's location. This is bound to a directed gaze and a defined field of vision. Against this background, close analogies can be found between schizophrenic speech disorders and those in pictorial

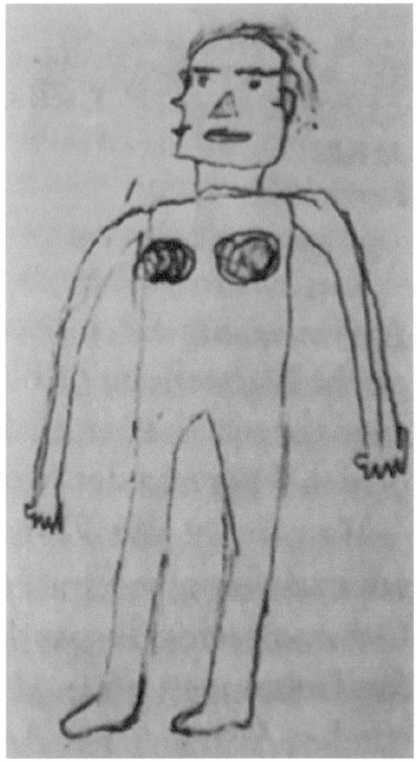

Fig. 4.15 Mixed profile with three eyes. A drawing by a patient with schizophrenia (Navratil, 1965, p. 79)

representation: Not mastering perspective and not recognizing the vanishing point is analogous to not recognizing the focus of the speech one is delivering. Phenomena such as derailment, concatenation, schizophasia, and the lack of perspective are manifestations of the same problem. The goal and the main theme of a speech are lost, as is the vanishing point in a composition without perspective (Figs. 4.15, 4.16, and 4.17).

Following the perspectival line is in a way like following the thread of conversation: Both intend to act logically and establish a purpose, a relationship, and a stringent connection between the different parts of a conversation or a graphic representation. Although the impairment of perspective in the figurative representation of individuals with schizophrenia is already evident from the analysis of earlier works, there are more specific illustrative examples. It is Leo Navratil again who offers some thought-provoking impulses:

> The partial fusion of a front view and a side view of a human head is called a mixed profile. [...] In the fusion of the front and the side view of the human head, a wealth of different combinations is possible. Most often (in works by individuals with schizophrenia, p.p.) one sees compositions in which two eyes are present, although the nose and mouth or one of the two details are already in profile position. In a mixed profile, the nose or the mouth can also be completely absent or presented twice, for example, one nose in front view and a second

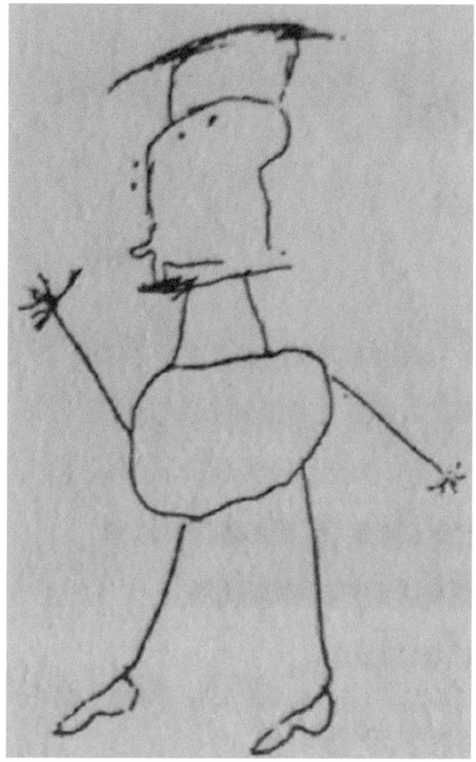

Fig. 4.16 Mixed profile with four eyes. A drawing by a patient with schizophrenia (Navratil, 1965, p. 80)

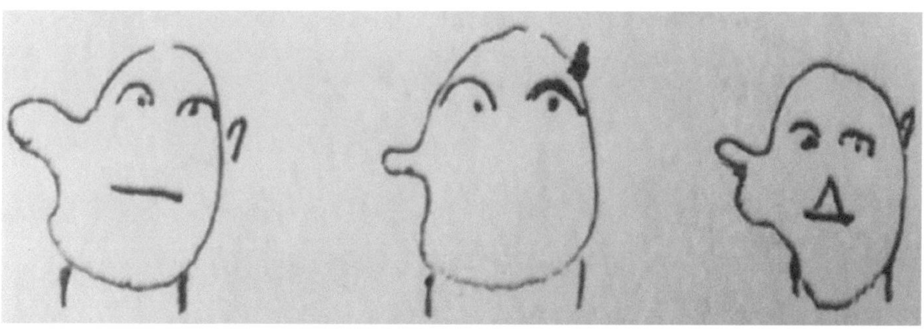

Fig. 4.17 Different forms of the mixed profile. Drawings by a patient with schizophrenia during the course of treatment (Navratil, 1965, p. 79)

in profile. Very rarely, when one detail is omitted, another is doubled. [...] Thus, in a drawing by a patient with schizophrenia we find the mouth twice, two noses, and three eyes; the profile eye lies in the contour of the face. The drawing of another patient with schizophrenia even shows four eyes, which, however, only appear as dots; the two profile eyes are outside the outline of the face, vertically one above the other; next to them are also a nose in profile and a displaced mouth *en face*. (Navratil, 1965, pp. 77–79; source in German)

The stylized drawings depict the people without any relationship to a surrounding space, without any attempt to create perspective.

In the drawings or paintings of individuals with schizophrenia, one can find various kinds of perspectival distortion, as can be observed in the drawings by young Franz and the colorful works by Livia Dencher (Landert, 2011, p. 118 f.) (Figs. 4.18 and 4.19).

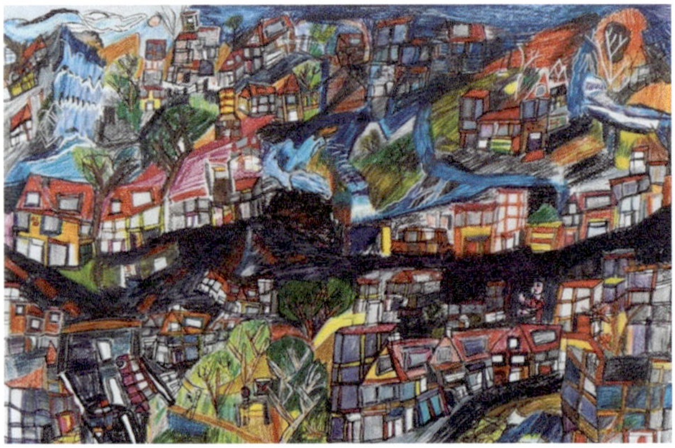

Fig. 4.18 Livia Dencher, *Untitled, 2009* (Landert, 2011, p. 118)

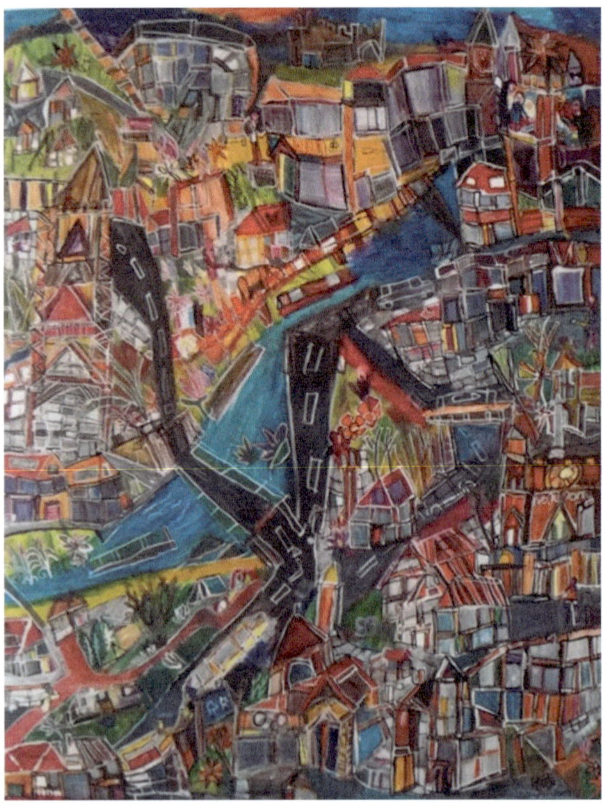

Fig. 4.19 Livia Dencher, *Frankrijk*, 2008 (Landert, 2011, p. 119)

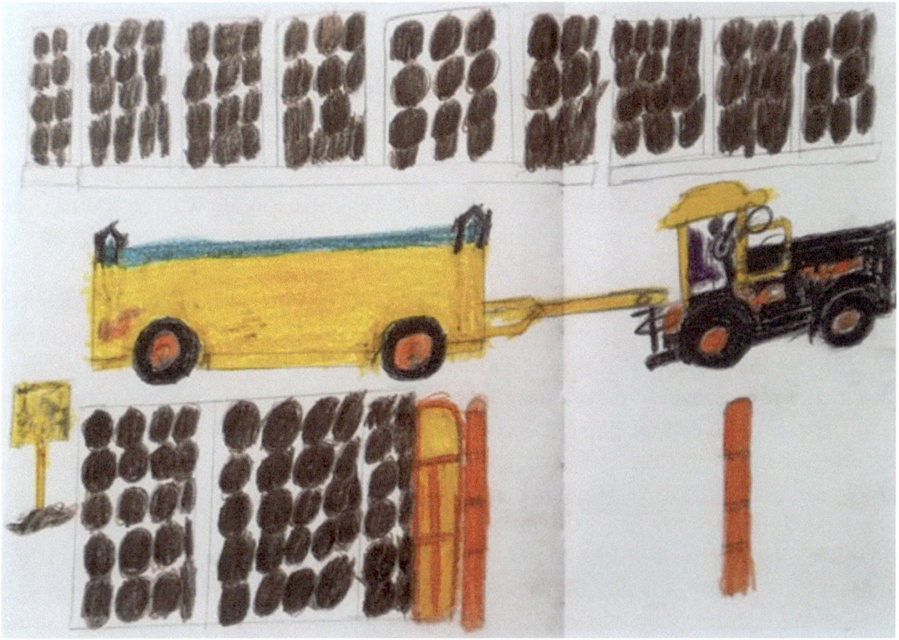

Fig. 4.20 Helmut Widmaier, *Untitled*, undated (Weber, 2008, pp. 44–45)

Another example of the copresence of different perspectives in one and the same figurative representation is offered by Helmut Widmeyer's drawing *Untitled* (Fig. 4.20). The horizontal middle section of the work offers a frontal perspective of a tractor, a trailer, and road sign. The upper and lower thirds of the drawing most likely provide an aerial perspective perpendicular to the frontal perspective. The position of the enigmatic brown spheres suggests that they are seen from top to bottom. Also that drawing is characterized by a lack of a unified spatial context. There is no uniformly directed view of the world, but many views, separate and side by side (Weber, 2008, p. 45).

Similarities between schizophrenic art and the pictures drawn by children have often been noted. These similarities are based on the fact that these images move far away from the objectifying paradigm of mimesis. This kind of perspective is called *affective perspective*. The size and dimensions of the depicted elements do not reflect the proportions of the theory of vision, but the affective, emotional, and inner resonance of the artist. Leo Navratil had recognized the importance of this fact:

> In children's drawings, similar in their way to some works of medieval art, the main characters are often depicted larger than the secondary characters, regardless of the spatial distance. Also, what is important to the child for some reason, for instance the hat on a human figure, can be drawn disproportionately large. Werner has termed this phenomenon the 'affect perspective' (Werner, 1953). In nature too, the size or smallness of an object often has a corresponding expressive value. However, this expressive value of relative size is distributed by the child according to its own needs, independently of the actual circum-

> stances. This process is mostly unconscious. Under affective influence, the perceptual content is transformed, which frequently leads to considerable disproportions. Individuals with schizophrenia often arbitrarily dispose of proportions in their drawings. The more prominent the feature of *disproportion* is, the more likely it is to be indicative of schizophrenia. In acute psychotic states, the drawings of patients with schizophrenia often show numerous disproportions. (Navratil, 1965, p. 100; source in German)

The drawing by Rosemarie Hübner (Fig. 4.21) corresponds well to the tile she had chosen. Apart from proportions, the affective meaning and relevance of the objects is also expressed here through colors.

Green is par excellence the color of spring. It is extremely abundant in Hübner's drawing leaving no room for sky and earth. One can speak of an *affective color perspective* that exists in addition to the previously described *affective perspective*, in which, for instance, objects are shown from several sides/perspectives at the same time. This affective color perspective works differently from the classical color perspective described in the Renaissance by Leonardo da Vinci. Flowers are the real and literal protagonists of Hübner's drawing, and one is even larger than the crudely depicted figure. Apart from the colorfulness, the other affective perspective that manifests itself in proportions also plays a role here. Twenty-nine flowers of different sizes and colors fill the entire space. The radiant sun smiles at the reborn and lush spring nature. The objects come to life and allow their emotions to shine through. This work, much like that of many children, is the triumph of emotions which turn into art. Here again one can observe some characteristics of artworks created by individuals with schizophrenia, such as, for instance, the *horror vacui (fear of empty spaces)* and the flattening without spatial depth.

Carlo Zinelli offers another interesting example of affective scale and affective color perspective (Fig. 4.22): The painting shows human figures and tiny characters filling in all the gaps between the forms (*horror vacui*). Two human silhouettes, presumably male because they appear to be wearing trousers, are the drawing's protagonists. Zinelli may have had a special relationship with these two figures

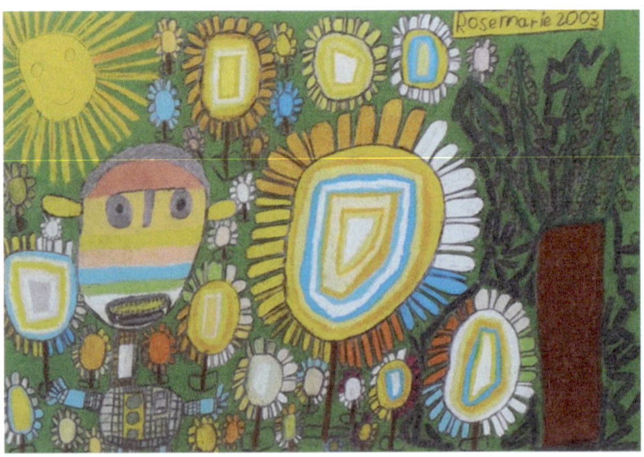

Fig. 4.21 Rosemarie Hübner, *Spring*, 2003 (Weber, 2008, p. 65)

Fig. 4.22 Carlo Zinelli, *People*, 1959 (Landert, 2011, p. 99)

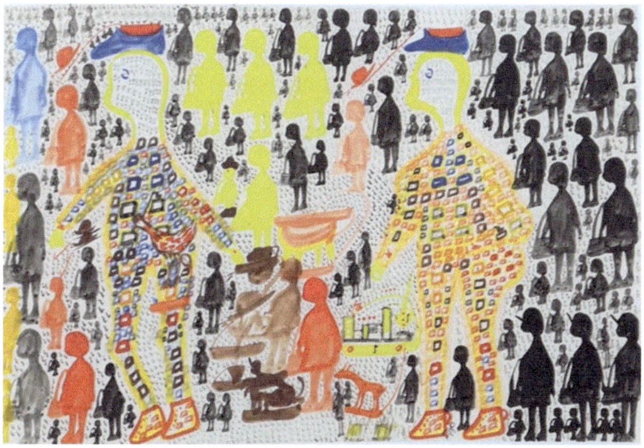

because they are large, and the affective perspective indicates greater emotional involvement on the part of the artist. The affective size relationships are matched by the affective color perspective. The two large figures appear in strikingly bright colors, while the small silhouettes surrounding the two large figures are colored in different ways: On the right side of the drawing, dark figures in shades of gray and black stand out, while in the center and on the left, dark silhouettes regularly alternate with light and primary-colored figures (yellow, red, blue). Since the silhouettes are almost identical, it can be argued that the main differences between them are given by size and color. The small figures of people are arranged over the entire field of the sheet without participating in a real three-dimensional space or being placed in a naturalistic environment. This work thus illustrates many peculiarities of schizophrenic painting.

4.5 Summary

Art and artistic expressions have features that can be explained in accordance with the *subjectivity-frame-perspective* theory as analogous to specific features of language behavior and micro-social behavior. This chapter has first suggested correlation between the manifestation of schizophrenia and the occurrence of a change in style through the analyses of clinical cases. Even though the patients and artists with schizophrenia show heterogeneous artistic styles with a tendency towards geometrization, repetition, and filling, for instance, a variety of forms, styles, and patterns can be observed that reveal the absence of perspective and the absence of frame. The artistic expressions of individuals with schizophrenia are often two-dimensional, and attempts at perspective often fail. The framelessness manifests itself not only in the absence of perspective correlated with it, but also in the inability to represent an a priori three-dimensional space. The depicted objects are simply juxtaposed, and even when an orderly composition is designed, as in the geometrizing and iterating style, for example, they are never located in a unified perceptual space created and opened by a depicting subject. The role of the subject as a center or as a standpoint from which a naturalistic and perspectival space can be represented is often absent in artistic expressions of individuals with schizophrenia. The absence of perspective and frame thus appears as an extreme form of a basic tendency of schizophrenic artistic expressions.

Analysis of Spatial Perception 5

5.1 Introduction

The perception of space has aroused the interest of philosophers and psychiatrists from the very beginning of the phenomenological tradition. The subjective perception of space is different from our understanding of space according to the principles and laws of mathematical physics. This chapter will provide a phenomenological analysis of the spatial perception in schizophrenia, based also on neuroscientific studies. Almost a century ago, Minkowski (1971, p. 386) first noticed the phenomenon of *macroscopy* in schizophrenia patients: Things are seen dimensionally larger than they would be normally perceived. Seeing objects larger or smaller than usual means that they are not perceived in a normal perspectival order, i.e., in a natural and uniform image or scene in which all things are proportionally arranged according to size and distance from the observer. Instead, they are perceived as objects in isolation, separated from any visual context or background. The phenomena of *macroscopy* and *microscopy* have not been studied as closely as other disorders of vision, on which most studies in the field of spatial perception focused on. The fragmentation of space and the difficulties that individuals with schizophrenia show in presenting space uniformly and in perspective have been analyzed in depth by neuropsychiatric researchers. This chapter presents the most significant findings regarding the altered perception of space in individuals with schizophrenia from the most recent studies.

5.2 Frame

To introduce this chapter that examines the various aspects of spatial perception in schizophrenia, I quote a page from the writer Peter Handke. He published a short story in 1970 entitled *Die Angst des Tormanns beim Elfmeter* (*The Goalkeeper's*

P. Parisi, *A Phenomenological Interpretation of Schizophrenia*,
https://doi.org/10.1007/978-3-031-67860-8_5

Anxiety at the Penalty Kick) (Handke, 1970), in which he vividly describes a psychotic state of the protagonist on the last pages of the book (Handke, 2020, pp. 83–84).

Handke's brilliant idea was to replace certain lexemes with iconic signs, i.e., schematic representations of things. The world appears fragmented, disintegrated, without a general frame. The protagonist, Bloch, sees the table, the glass, the cupboard, the bed, the suitcase, the match, and all the other objects that present themselves to him as separated entities, indeed only as schemata. Handke expresses the spatial relationships between the objects through adverbs of place but indicates the objects themselves with icons. A few lines further, the author dispenses entirely with punctuation marks. The various objects are juxtaposed, and there is not even a comma to relate the different objects to one another.

Handke presents how fragmented the world is perceived by the protagonist during his psychosis. Bloch shows an utterly impaired spatial perception. Regardless of whether it is in fact schizophrenia that we are dealing with or another form of mental disorder, this description is relevant because it illustrates the *loosening of associations* (cf. Bleuler, 1911) and the loss of the ability to take an objective and holistic viewpoint.

5.2.1 The Problem of Global Vision

Many studies conducted in recent years in order to investigate the way individuals with schizophrenia would perceive space have suggested quite specific patterns of visual perception. The problem these patients seem to have is integrating visual information into an overall picture or *Gestalt*. The various experiments that have been carried out and will be presented in the following show that individuals with schizophrenia tend to focus on specific details instead of perceiving the scene holistically as a whole.

5.2.2 Global Scanning

As has already been mentioned, the perception of an overall picture is impaired in individuals with schizophrenia, and the way in which they scan the visual field with their eyes has been studied extensively over the last 30 years. Gordon, for example, was the first to observe how individuals with schizophrenia scan a face as they gaze upon a person. Unlike non-schizophrenic subjects who focus their attention on the nose, eyes, and cheeks (Walker-Smith et al., 1977, pp. 313–326), individuals with schizophrenia look at fewer fixation points and therefore miss salient areas of the face (Gordon et al., 1992, pp. 626–629; Streit et al., 1997, pp. 311–317).

Impaired visual scanning modalities have also been noted when observing schizophrenia patients in social settings. Again, neurophysiological studies have confirmed that patients with schizophrenia often do not observe the social environment as a whole.[1] This consequently implies a limitation in their dealings with social situations (Williams et al., 2003, pp. 13–27). The visual patterning of individuals with schizophrenia is altered (less visual fixation and smaller observed scanning area) even when they look at images that do not depict social scenes (Green et al., 2000, pp. 63–74; Hahn et al., 2012, pp. 119–128; Kojima et al., 1992, pp. 85–94; Ryu et al., 2001, pp. 369–376), as in the case of the Rorschach test (Minassian et al., 2005, pp. 69–79).

The study by Bestelmeyer et al. (2006, pp. 212–222) is a synthesis of what had previously been analyzed by other researchers. Bestelmeyer et al. examined the visual patterns of 22 patients with schizophrenia and compared these with 37 non-schizophrenic subjects. The subjects were given 28 color photographs of faces, landscapes, fractals, and pink dot compositions and were requested to look at each image freely and spontaneously. In addition, participants could also request a break during the experiment if they felt they needed one. The total duration of the experiment was 15 min on average.

The eye movements are displayed on each image (Fig. 5.1). The size of the circles is proportional to the fixation time of the image. The larger the circle, the longer the fixation time. The analysis shows two major differences between individuals with schizophrenia and the control group: Non-schizophrenic subjects tend to focus on all areas first and grasp the content. They spend relatively little time on details. Individuals with schizophrenia, on the other hand, have longer fixation times and a narrower viewing area. Unlike the non-schizophrenic individuals, however, individuals with schizophrenia do not seem to grasp the totality of the picture, and furthermore, they do not attempt to outline and integrate the various elements of the representation with their gaze. This impairment is evident as regards all types of image and does not only apply to faces or landscape photographs. In line with the above studies, it can be concluded that there is a general impairment of global vision in individuals with schizophrenia.

5.2.3 Global Vs. Local

According to Navon's global precedence theory, physiologically, the processing of visual information shows a preference of moving from the global to the local level. Navon's original study reveals how the act of seeing proceeds from global to local (Navon, 1977, pp. 353–383). Navon's conclusion has been confirmed in the findings

[1] Gaebel et al. (1987, pp. 1227–1237), Loughland et al. (2002, pp. 159–170), Manor and Gordon (2003, pp. 85–93), Phillips and David (1997, pp. 99–105), Phillips and David (1998, pp. 235–245), Williams et al. (1999, pp. 189–199).

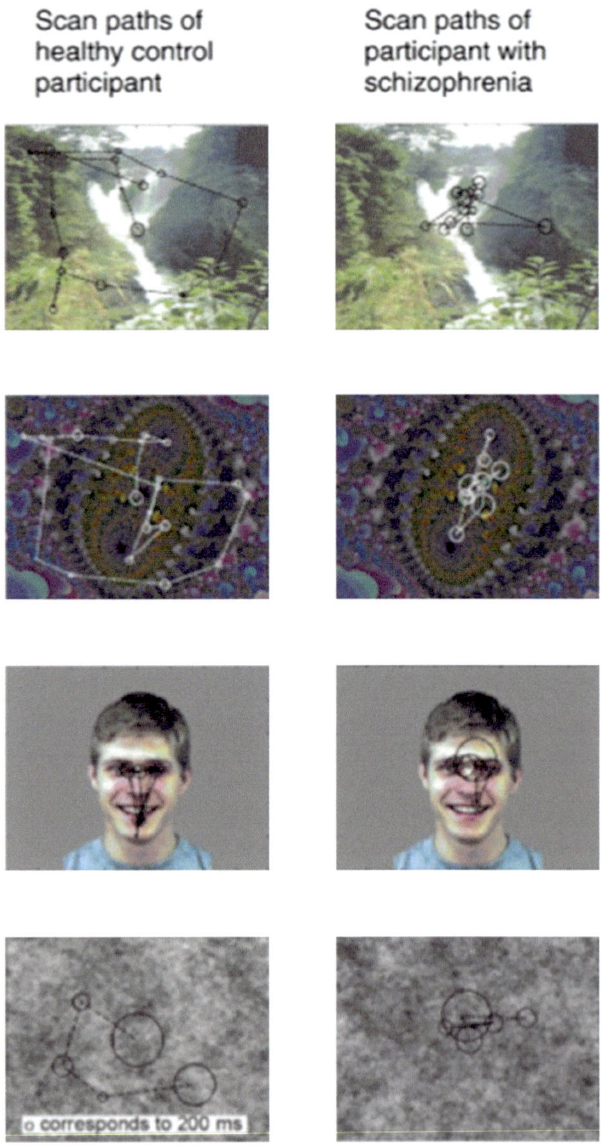

Fig. 5.1 Comparison between visual scanning of images in non-schizophrenic (healthy) and in subjects with schizophrenia (Bestelmeyer et al., 2006, p. 217)

of subsequent studies summarized in Kimchi's article (Kimchi, 1992, pp. 24–38). Many studies have also been conducted on the lateralization of the right or left hemisphere of the brain in order to investigate how global or local visual information is processed, respectively.[2]

[2]Delis et al. (1988, pp. 421–431), Evans (2000, pp. 225–239), Fink et al. (1996, pp. 626–628), Heinze et al. (1998, pp. 485–498), Lamb and Robertson (1988, pp. 172–181), Martinez et al. (1997, pp. 1437–1457), Proverbio et al. (1998, pp. 321–334), van Kleeck (1989, pp. 1165–1178), Weber et al. (2000, pp. 241–247).

The results showed that the patients' processing of local stimuli is better than the processing of global stimuli.

Based on results from the eye movement studies and on the assumption that individuals with schizophrenia prefer the particular or local view to the general or global view, Landgraf and colleagues conducted a study to support this thesis (Landgraf et al., 2011, pp. 163–170). In this experiment, 24 individuals with schizophrenia and 25 non-schizophrenic subjects were given the *mental mirroring task*, and the eye movements of the two groups were recorded.

In this task, the study subjects were presented with certain pairs of patterns of squares between which there are mirror-image relationships: (**a**) identical, (**b**) vertical, (**c**) horizontal, or (**d**) diagonal (Fig. 5.2). The participants were asked to complete a total of 4 blocks, each consisting of 12 pairs of patterns. The experiment consisted of finding the six pairs in each block between which there was a mirror relationship and the six pairs between which there was no mirror relationship.

The results of this experiment confirmed findings from previous neurophysiological studies and showed that individuals with schizophrenia process local rather than global visual stimuli (Cavezian et al., 2007, pp. 257–264; Parnas et al., 2001 pp. 171–180; Dreben et al., 1995, pp. 447–465; Johnson et al., 2005, pp. 937–946). Landgraf and his colleagues concluded that:

1. Task difficulty influences patients' deficits. Patients show increased reaction time under the easiest conditions and elevated error rates under the more difficult conditions compared to healthy controls.
2. Information processing mediates patients' deficits. Patients show similar fixation duration under all four conditions of difficulty, whereas healthy controls adapt their mean fixation duration to the demands of the task.
3. Under the easiest condition, patients rely on short fixations and more on long fixations compared to healthy controls. This pattern tends to reverse under the most difficult condition.
4. Negative symptoms correlated with fixation duration in the identity condition.
5. Medication intake did not correlate with any of the tasks' measures (Landgraf et al., 2011, p. 167).

In the second study conducted by Johnson and his colleagues (Johnson et al., 2005, pp. 937–946), two groups were studied and compared: The group of individuals with schizophrenia consisted of 24 subjects (14 men, 10 women) and the group of non-schizophrenic subjects consisted of 29 subjects (15 men, 14 women). The age of the individuals with schizophrenia ranged from 15 to 66 years and that of the non-schizophrenic subjects from 19 to 69 years.

The participants were asked to pay close attention to the letters E, T, H, and U (only three types of letters are shown in the example). As can be seen above (Fig. 5.3), each capital letter is composed of smaller letters, which creates two levels—one global and one local. Participants were given the information that a letter will be displayed on a computer screen, and they were requested to perform the following task: Each time they perceived an H, they had to press a specific key with their right index finger. In

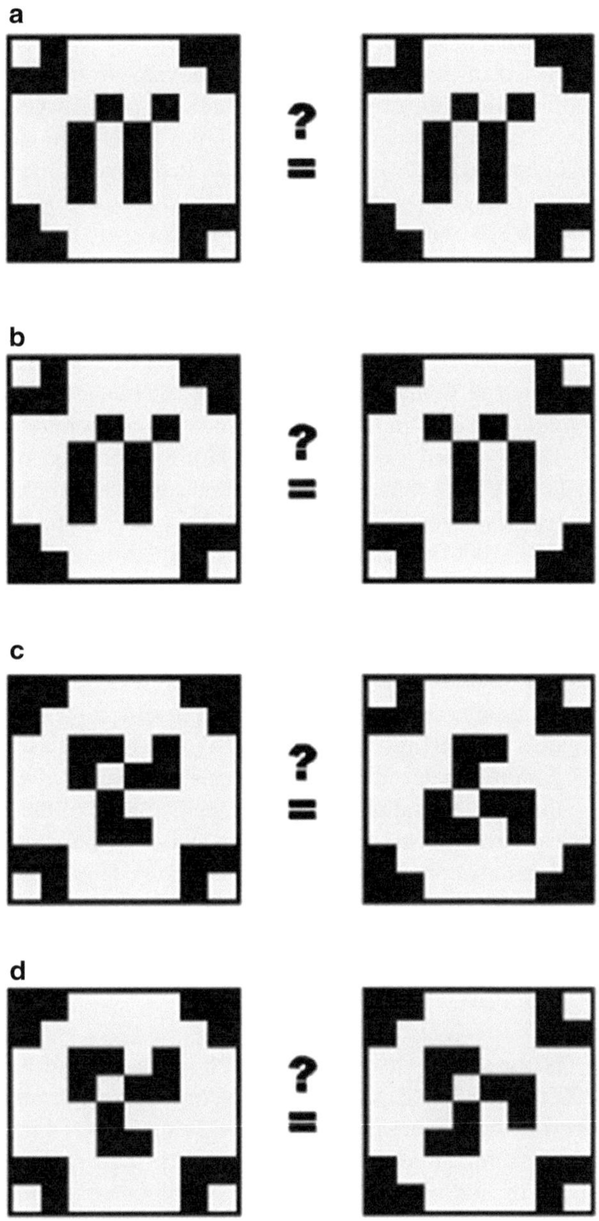

Fig. 5.2 Examples of the pattern recognition task (**a**–**d**). The task consisted of four blocks, and the following properties had to be recognized: (**a**) equality, (**b**) vertical mirroring, (**c**) horizontal mirroring, (**d**) diagonal mirroring (Landgraf et al., 2011, p. 165)

the experiment, the letter H appeared both locally and globally. In total, 240 stimuli were presented in random order: 60 at the global level, 60 at the local level, and 120 distractors (in the example, the letter T is formed by the smaller letters U where the letter H does not actually appear). In order to familiarize the participants with the experiment, five tests were carried out in advance as a practice exercise.

```
E   E      HHHHH      UUUUU
E   E      H            U
EEEEE      HHHH         U
E   E      H            U
E   E      HHHHH        U

GLOBAL 'H'  LOCAL 'H'  DISTRACTOR
```

Fig. 5.3 Examples of local and global stimuli. The task concerns the recognition of an H without specifying whether this is local or global (Johnson et al., 2005, p. 938)

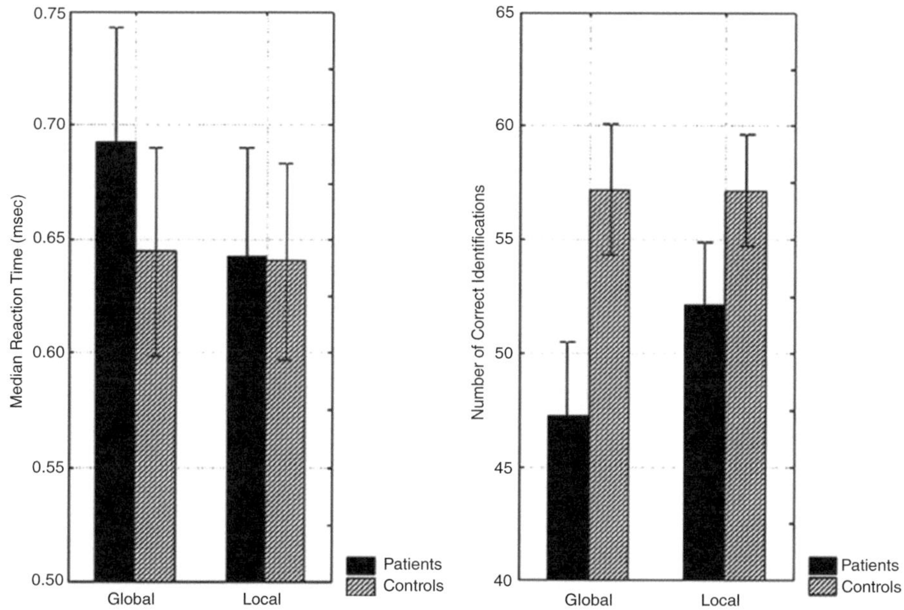

Fig. 5.4 Result of the comparison between patients with schizophrenia and non-schizophrenic subjects (controls) (Johnson et al., 2005, p. 941)

The results (Fig. 5.4) show interesting differences between the two groups. In the graph on the left, it can be observed that the reaction time to a local stimulus does not differ between the two groups, while the reaction time to a global stimulus is significantly longer in the group of individuals with schizophrenia. These patients give more incorrect responses, as can be seen in the graph on the right. It can also be observed that the greatest difference between correct and incorrect responses in the two groups is in the recognition of signs at the global level.

Another study, conducted by Kurylo and his colleagues, approached the deficit of individuals with schizophrenia in visual perception in a different way. The aim of the study (Kurylo et al., 2007, pp. 205–214) was to determine the ability of individuals with schizophrenia to organize visual perception. The study participants were divided into two groups: 19 patients with schizophrenia (17 male and 2 female) and 20 non-schizophrenic individuals (11 male and 9 female).

They were shown lines formed by white dots on a black background on a screen (Fig. 5.5a) and requested to determine whether these lines were horizontal or vertical. In some images, the dots formed very clear lines, while in other images the dots were so far apart from each other that no clear lines could be discerned. To decide whether the lines were horizontal or vertical was not a problem for the study participants as long as the dots in the lines were close enough to one another and the distances between the lines larger. In the second part of the experiment, horizontal or vertical lines of green and red dots were presented (Fig. 5.5b). The lines appear clear to perceive when lines of red dots alternate with lines of green dots; however, the lines become indistinguishable when a line is formed by both, red and green dots.

The results of the experiment show a significant difference between the individuals with schizophrenia and the control group of non-schizophrenic subjects: In the first part of the experiment, the individuals with schizophrenia needed the white dots to be closer to each other in order to recognize the lines, and in the second part of the experiment, the lines had to have a more uniform color to be recognized as lines by the patients with schizophrenia.

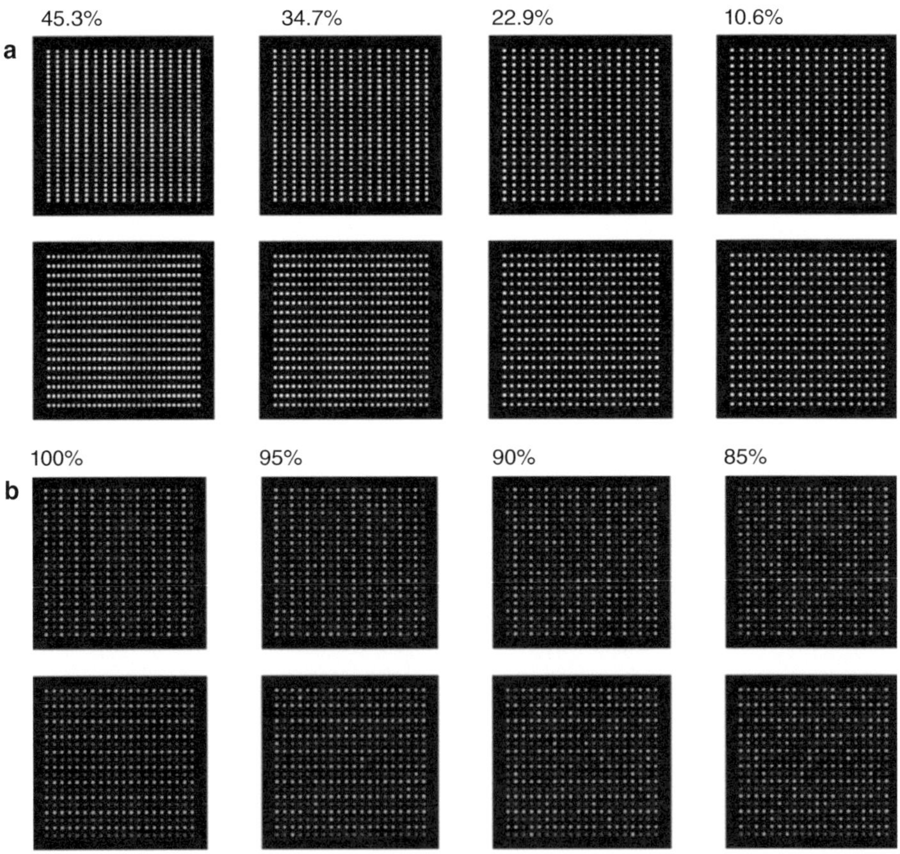

Fig. 5.5 Examples of spatial and chromatic proximity (**a**, **b**) (Kurylo et al., 2007, p. 208)

The authors of the study regard these results (Fig. 5.6) as further experimental evidence of the fact that individuals with schizophrenia are more impaired in processing global stimuli.

The complex relationship between local and global visual perception can also be approached from another perspective. Neurocognitive studies have shown that people tend to see concise shapes even if they are not complete. When a form is a familiar one, it is reconstructed, even if the visual stimuli are incomplete (Doniger et al., 2001, pp. 305–313; Murray et al., 2002, pp. 5055–5073).

Ikeda et al. (2011, pp. 231–238) conducted a test with 20 patients with schizophrenia between the ages of 17 and 49 and 20 non-schizophrenic subjects of similar average age. The four figures in Fig. 5.7 show four different stimuli:

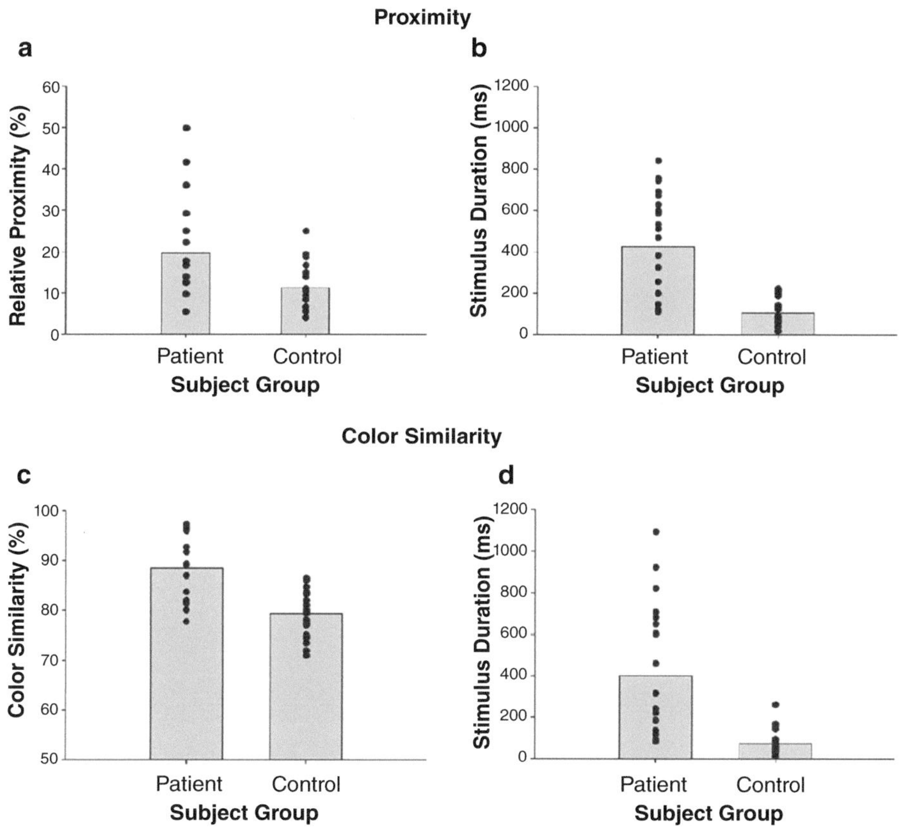

Fig. 5.6 Result of the comparison between patients with schizophrenia and non-schizophrenic (control) subjects. Performance for (**a**) proximity grouping thresholds, (**b**) proximity-critical stimulus duration for perceptual grouping, (**c**) color similarity grouping thresholds, and (**d**) color similarity-critical stimulus duration. Each circle represents an individual subject. The bars show the group mean (Kurylo et al., 2007, p. 210)

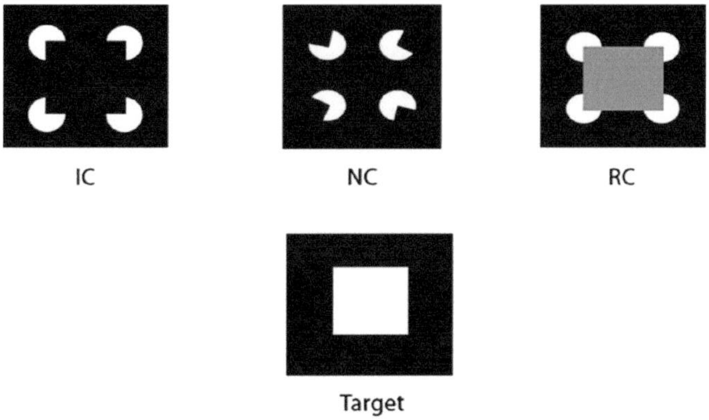

Fig. 5.7 Kanizsa square. Stimulus categories (Ikeda et al., 2011, p. 233)

1. IC = Illusory contour (or Kanizsa square)
2. NC = No contour
3. RC = Real contour
4. Target

The non-schizophrenic subjects and the patients with schizophrenia were shown four stimuli. The P100 latency in individuals with schizophrenia to recognize IC was longer than in non-schizophrenic subjects (Ikeda et al., 2011, p. 231).

The authors concluded:

> The present findings revealed that processing of IC in schizophrenia might be specifically deteriorated and associated with the clinical symptoms of the disease. (Ikeda et al., 2011, p. 236)

Recognizing an illusory contour, such as Kanizsa square, means being able to integrate different elements of the same composition in such a way as to complete the parts of a negative profile into a concise figure. This study suggests that the processing of global visual perception is impaired in individuals with schizophrenia, since this task proved impossible for the patients.

5.2.4 Global Symmetry

The visual perception of local or global dimensions was investigated by further studies on the perception of symmetry. A composition of elements is symmetrical if the elements are equidistant from an axis of symmetry. The presence of an axis of symmetry implies recognition of the composition as a unit. The elements of a symmetrical composition are therefore not symmetrical by virtue of themselves but by virtue of their relation to each other. Although it may hardly seem evident at first glance, the frame plays the central role here as the guarantor of the general order of the composition. The frame has a superordinate function. An axis of symmetry can only become an axis of symmetry in relation to a frame.

Recently, many neurophysiological and behavioral studies have been developed on the recognition of symmetries. It has been found that for non-schizophrenic subjects it is easier to notice and to remember (in short-term memory) symmetries on vertical axes than any other type of symmetry or asymmetry (Imbo et al., 2009, pp. 275–291; Kemps, 2001, pp. 13–27; Pieroni et al., 2011, pp. 145–159; Rossi-Arnaud et al., 2006, pp. 393–400). Anthropologically, this could be a consequence of the upright gait adopted in the course of evolution.

In this context, the study by Cestari et al. (2013, pp. 594–603) is worth mentioning. The study was conducted with 20 patients with schizophrenia recruited in the San Giovanni Evangelista hospital in Tivoli and 20 non-schizophrenic subjects of similar average age. This experiment is similar to that of Landgraf et al. (2011); however, here the focus is on short-term memory and a greater attention is required. In addition, Cestari's study was more complex and aimed at investigating the possible impairment in schizophrenia in remembering symmetrical compositions at different levels.

The study subjects were presented with 96 patterns with different axes of symmetry (Fig. 5.8). Each pattern consisted of 25 squares (each 2 × 2 cm) arranged in 5 rows of 5. The 96 patterns were divided into 4 groups (24 asymmetrical, 24 vertically symmetrical, 24 horizontally symmetrical, and 24 diagonally symmetrical). In each of these four groups, there are patterns made of different numbers of colored squares (minimum 2, maximum 9) and of different difficulty. The participants were instructed to memorize the location of the red squares (here grey). Each test began with the presentation of a dot on a screen for 500 ms, followed by the presentation of the squares pattern for 3 s. Then, after a break of 2 s with a white screen, the participants had to remember the pattern that had been displayed to them.

The aim of the study was not only to find out which group made more mistakes but also what kind of mistakes occurred (Fig. 5.9). Therefore, not only a quantitative but also a qualitative evaluation was carried out.

The following graph (Fig. 5.10) shows that patients with schizophrenia gave fewer correct answers than non-schizophrenic subjects in all four pattern groups. While the recall of vertical symmetries was better in both groups, the asymmetrical patterns were most poorly remembered by both groups.

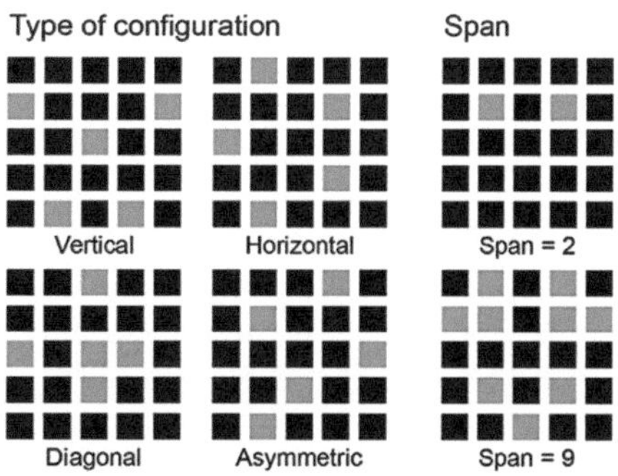

Fig. 5.8 Examples of symmetrical and asymmetrical compositions. In the experiment, the gray elements were red. *Span* refers to the number of red (here grey) squares (Cestari et al., 2013, p. 596)

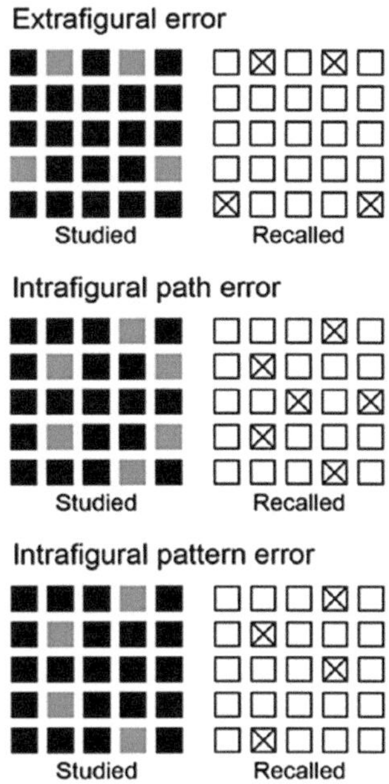

Fig. 5.9 Examples of incorrect answers (Cestari et al., 2013, p. 597)

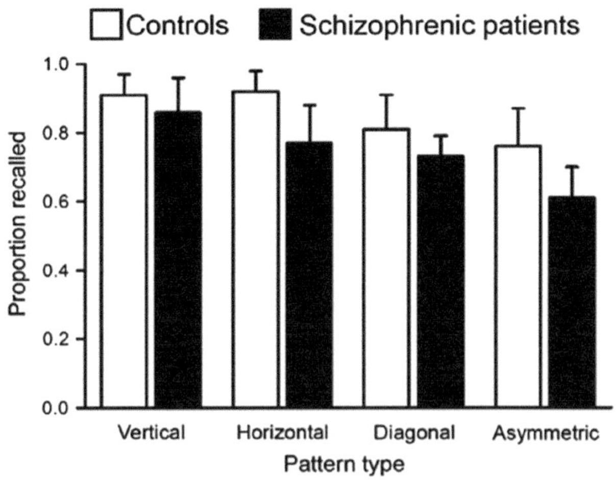

Fig. 5.10 Graph of the overall results (Cestari et al., 2013, p. 597)

As to the patterns with symmetries (Fig. 5.11), the following can be observed:

(a) Overall, the group of individuals with schizophrenia performed worse than the control group.
(b) As the difficulty of the task increased, individuals with schizophrenia had a greater deficit of correct answers than non-schizophrenic individuals.
(c) The non-schizophrenic subjects also had the most difficulties with diagonally symmetrical tasks, although to a slightly lesser extent than the individuals with schizophrenia.

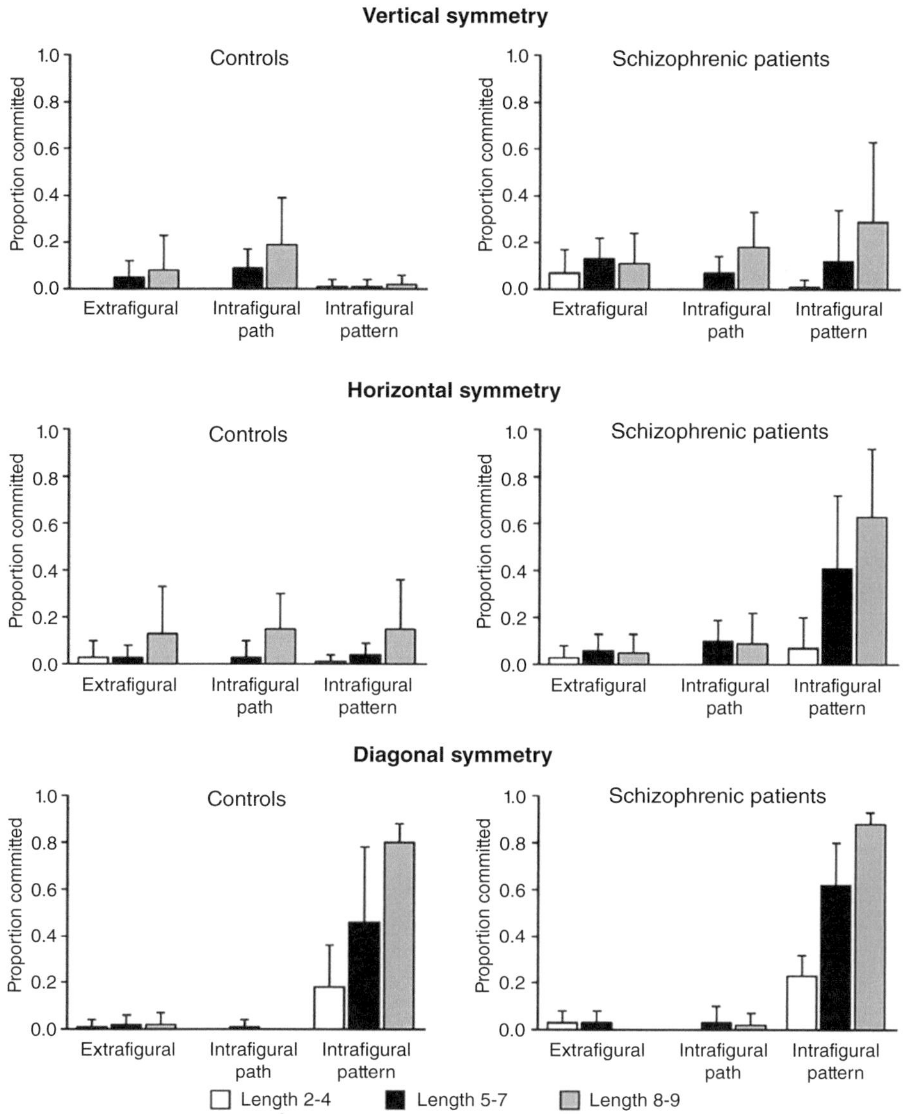

Fig. 5.11 Graph of the specific results (Cestari et al., 2013, p. 600)

This study is in line with previous data from the scientific literature, which showed that non-schizophrenic subjects can recall vertically symmetrical structures best. Furthermore, individuals with schizophrenia are worse at dealing with complex visual information (global stimulation) where short-term memory plays a role.

5.3 Perspective

5.3.1 Egocentrism Vs. Allocentrism

Video games have experienced great progress in recent years, and 3D representations are becoming better and more realistic. The landscapes, roads, paths, and other features of the natural and urban environment are so capable of drawing the viewer into the scenery that many children and young people are "hypnotized" by virtual games and thus transported into their virtual reality. Neuroscientists have used these new technologies to examine how the brains of non-schizophrenic individuals and the brains of people with schizophrenia respond to such visual stimuli (Amorim, 2003, pp. 157–199; Lambrey et al., 2008, pp. 523–534; Schmidt et al., 2007, pp. 955–968; Vogeley et al., 2004, pp. 817–827).

The key terms of the experiments conducted in this field are *allocentrism* and *egocentrism*. The term *allocentrism* is defined as the ability to orient oneself in the space surrounding the individual by means of objects, persons, or reference points. *Egocentrism* refers to a perspective that is experienced idiosyncratically by the subject.

The data available in the international scientific literature show an impairment of the allocentric perspective in subjects with schizophrenia, while the egocentric spatial orientation remains intact. The experiments performed by Langdon et al. (2001, pp. 241–269) and Agarwal et al. (2015, pp. 304-311) support this theory:

> The allocentric-egocentric dichotomy is of special relevance in schizophrenia: The allocentric simulation hypothesis postulates that the pathological referencing in schizophrenia is due to a problem in adopting a 'world-centred'—inter-subjective—reference frame. (Agarwal et al., 2017, pp. 276–277)

Impairment in visuospatial orientation in individuals with schizophrenia corresponds to their deficits in social relationships, empathy, and the ability to take on the perspective of others, as described by the *theory of mind* (Bosia et al., 2012, pp. 2284–2304; Decety & Lamm, 2007, pp. 580–593; Iacoboni & Dapretto, 2006, pp. 942–951; Thakkar & Park, 2010, pp. 477–500).

Neurophysiological studies suggest that the hippocampus and the medial structures of the temporal lobe are responsible for allocentric orientation abilities, while the striatal and parietal regions correlate with egocentrism (Burgess et al., 2001, pp. 625–641; Etchamendy & Bohbot, 2007, pp. 595–599; Zhang et al. 2013, pp. 1070–1087).

Two significant studies were conducted on allocentrism and egocentrism in schizophrenic individuals.

The first study dates from 2007 and was published a year later by Weniger and Irle (2008, pp. 201–209). 25 individuals with schizophrenia were compared with 25 non-schizophrenic subjects performing two different orientation tasks in virtual reality. The test consisted of two tasks that took place in different virtual scenarios. In one task, a realistic environment (landscape) was shown; in the other a path between walls without objective reference points (i.e., maze). Being in a landscape means being spatially confronted with houses, trees, clearly defined paths, cars, bridges, rivers, lakes, mountains, or clear reference points on the horizon. The maze, on the other hand, has none of that: The stones forming the walls of the maze all appear the same.

While the maze in Fig. 5.12a stimulates navigation and self-centered orientation, Fig. 5.12c stimulates allocentric orientation based on objective reference points in the environment outside the subject.

The test participants were shown a three-dimensional, colored, and detailed representation of a spatial environment (landscape or maze) and controlled their movements in that space using a joystick. The two virtual reality tasks were repeated five times over by each participant. On each path through the maze and the landscape, there is a container, but only one contains money. The participants' task was to find the fastest and most direct way to the container with the money. At the beginning of each repetition, all participants always started from the same starting point. The perspective of the aerial view of both the maze and landscape and the maze (Fig. 5.12b, d) was not presented to the subjects. Thus, during the task the only possible perspective was the first-person perspective. The aerial perspective could only be constructed from experience gained by each subject.

The results were: In the spatial orientation task in the landscape, most subjects reported that they had memorized environmental points (non-schizophrenic

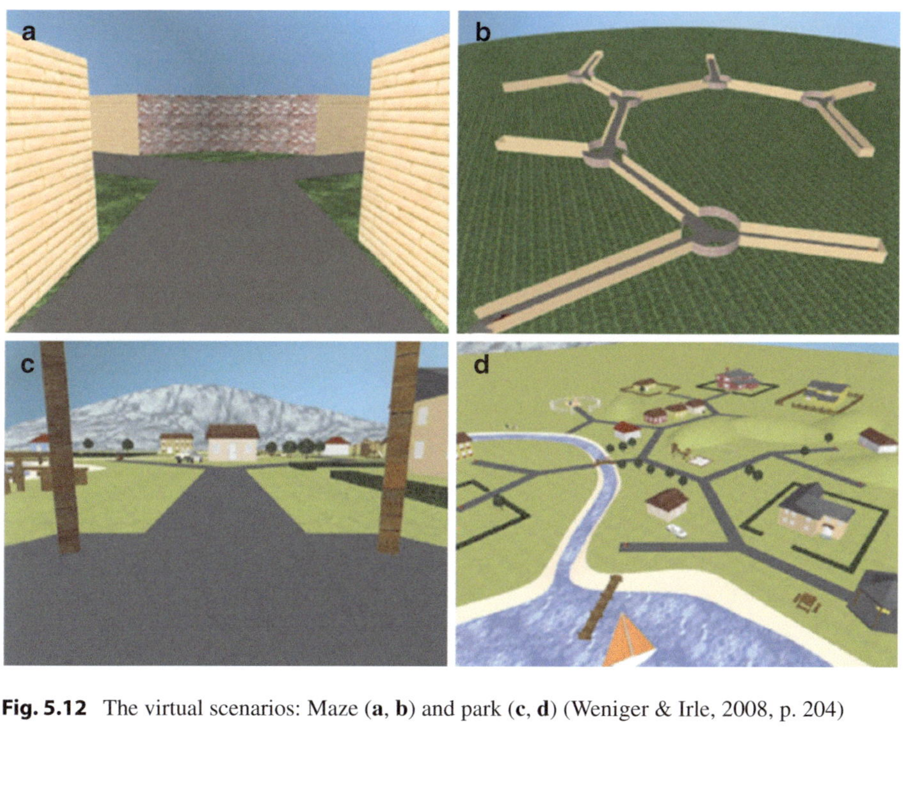

Fig. 5.12 The virtual scenarios: Maze (**a**, **b**) and park (**c**, **d**) (Weniger & Irle, 2008, p. 204)

subjects: 76%; subjects with schizophrenia: 59%), constructed an aerial perspective (non-schizophrenic subjects: 14%; subjects with schizophrenia: 9%), and remembered egocentric, i.e., body-related cues (non-schizophrenic subjects: 5%; subjects with schizophrenia: 18%). 5% of the non-schizophrenic individuals and 14% of the individuals with schizophrenia reported that they had not used any specific orientation strategy.

In the spatial orientation task in the maze, most subjects reported that they had memorized egocentric landmarks (non-schizophrenic subjects: 42%; subjects with schizophrenia: 52%) and the aerial perspective (non-schizophrenic subjects: 43%; subjects with schizophrenia: 24%). 14% of the non-schizophrenic subjects and 24% of the individuals with schizophrenia reported that they had not used any orientation strategy.

The graph above (Fig. 5.13) shows that for individuals with schizophrenia, it is more difficult to orient themselves in the landscape (allocentric perspective) than in the maze (egocentric perspective), where their results are even slightly better than those of the control group of non-schizophrenic subjects. The sign # indicates a significant difference between the two groups (t-test; $P < 0.001$).

Weniger and Irle conclude:

> Our results demonstrate a strong impairment of schizophrenia subjects to learn their way in a virtual park rich of navigationally relevant landmarks. [...] To our knowledge, the present study is the first to investigate egocentric navigation and memory storage of schizophrenia subjects in a virtual maze lacking any topographical landmarks. Compared with controls, the performance of schizophrenia subjects appeared entirely normal. Schizophrenia subjects more often reported to have used egocentric navigation strategies than controls, underlining the unimpaired egocentric navigation and memory processes of these subjects. The result is even more astonishing, as control subjects had more difficulties in learning the virtual maze compared with the virtual park. (Weniger & Irle, 2008, p. 206).

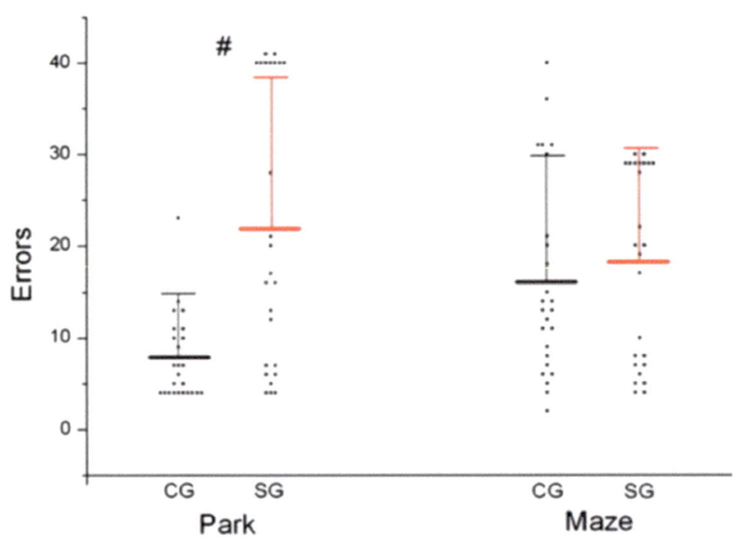

Fig. 5.13 Errors made in the virtual landscape and virtual maze (Weniger & Irle, 2008, p. 204)

The second study dates from 2017 and was conducted by a group of Iranian researchers from Tehran Medical University (Mohammadi et al., 2017, pp. 1–18). The purpose of the study was the same as in the first study, but in addition bipolar patients were also introduced here for comparison. The study involved a total of 60 participants (20 individuals with schizophrenia, 20 subjects with a bipolar disorder, and 20 healthy control subjects) who underwent two spatial orientation and memory tasks under egocentric and allocentric perspectives, respectively (Fig. 5.14).

The two-dimensional aerial representations were only presented at the beginning of the task for a duration of 60 s. A yellow circle on the photograph represented the goal of the orientation task: In the urban landscape, the task was to find a parking space and in the maze a sphere.

Before the start of the actual test, the participants were allowed three practice tests.

The results of the study by Mohammadi and colleagues (Fig. 5.15) confirmed the deficit of individuals with schizophrenia in spatial orientation based on an allocentric perspective. The data collected in the experiment also revealed a significant impairment in patients with schizophrenia in egocentric orientation. The subjects with a bipolar disorder showed no significant differences in comparison with the control group.

This review of the literature confirms that individuals with schizophrenia present impairments in the ability of three-dimensional spatial orientation to varying degrees and in different modalities. They have a greater deficit in the allocentric perspective than in the egocentric perspective. The degree of impairment in spatial orientation correlates with the severity of the clinical features. Patients with schizophrenia often orient themselves from an egocentric perspective. This can be explained by the fact that the allocentric perspective is impaired because the subject obviously does not have a secure point of view and the spatial perception associated with it is too loose. The necessary condition for an allocentric perspective is a firm, clear, and distinct relationship between the subject and the object, which will be discussed in more detail further on.

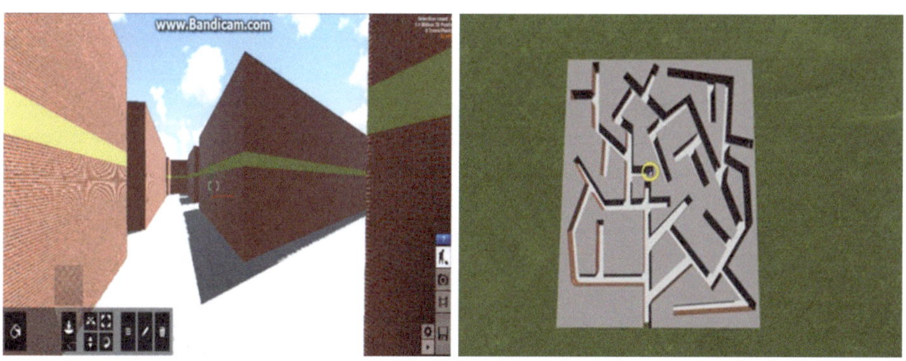

Fig. 5.14 Egocentric and allocentric perspective (Mohammadi et al., 2017, p. 6)

Patients	Allocentric	Egocentric
Schizophrenia	Impaired[a] (Getting lost and confused in navigation)	Impaired[a] (Better performance than allocentric, Longer response time than allocentric and confused in navigation)
Bipolar disorder	Almost not impaired[b] (Little confused in navigation)	Almost not impaired[b] (Better performance than allocentric and longer response time than allocentric)

[a]Significantly lower than normal subjects.
[b]Slightly lower than normal subjects, but not significant.

Fig. 5.15 Results of the study by Mohammadi et al. (2017)

5.3.2 Concave or Convex

To perceive the world in a perspectival way means to include depth of field. Photographers, directors, painters, and other artists know this well. Twentieth-century art provides a large number of examples in which depth of field is absent: James Turrell's light installations that present only pure color, i.e., colored light, are a prime example of this (Kim, 2013; Reed, 2019; Schürmann, 1998). The visual pyramid of perspective construction offers a concave space in the sense that the perspectival vanishing point is on the horizon and in front of the viewer, who can enter into the space because it originally appears to him or her as deep and open. Such a perspectival perception arises from the dimensions of objects that become smaller on their way to the vanishing point.

Perspectival vision is the prerequisite for the perception of concave and convex shapes.

Throughout the history of art and science, there has been much experimentation with optical illusions. Among the most interesting of these illusions that play with three-dimensionality and concave or convex perception is the so-called hollow face illusion (or hollow mask illusion, Gregory, 1970): The mask appears convex both when presented to the viewer from the convex side and when presented to him or her from the concave side. It is assumed that the human brain automatically corrects the perception of the mask by adapting the perception to the usual and accustomed perceptual world in which human faces only appear convex. The hollow face illusion is part of a group of tests that have been able to show experimentally that, for example, physically convex objects are perceived as concave due to the assumed habitual perception and vice versa.

Hollow mask illusion tests had been performed with individuals with schizophrenia and show that they often do not fall for optical illusions, as is normally the case with non-schizophrenic individuals, but that they perceive correctly according to the presentation of the hollow mask (Dima et al., 2009, pp. 1180–1186; Dima et al., 2010, pp. 824–832; Emrich, 1989, pp. 37–39; Rohleder et al., 2018; Schneider et al., 1996, pp. 256–260; Schneider et al., 2002, pp. 101–108). It has also been shown that the illusion provoked in perspectival reversal tests was significantly less frequent in people with an altered consciousness resulting from cannabinoid consumption (Emrich et al., 1991, pp. 689–690; Leweke et al., 1999, pp. 230–235; Leweke et al., 2000, pp. 175–181; Semple et al., 2003, pp. 789–793). Thus, parallels between the state of consciousness in schizophrenia and the state after cannabinoid consumption can be observed.

Steven Silverstein, Thomas Papathomas, and their colleagues have developed an important experiment, which is part of *depth inversion illusions* (DIIs), in order to test perspectival visual perception in individuals with schizophrenia.

The first study (Keane et al., 2013, pp. 506–512) was conducted in 2013 involving 30 patients with schizophrenia and 25 control subjects. The participants were presented with two masks, both concave, one in a homogeneous shade of beige and the other with painted facial features. Both masks were concave, but non-schizophrenic subjects tended to see them as convex. To ensure that participants did not respond randomly to the perceived convexity or concavity of the mask, the researchers also introduced a physically convex mask to monitor the perception. In addition to the two concave masks and the convex mask, two horizontally oriented convex truncated pyramids were presented facing the observer which, however, were perceived physiologically and for perspectival reasons as concave. One pyramid appeared in a homogenous beige tone, the other was painted with naturalistic environmental features (Fig. 5.16).

One can understand better the construction of the truncated pyramids and the illusion they create, thanks to a YouTube video uploaded by the scientists (https://www.youtube.com/watch?v=BlKlpx50Avs). The illusion of the hollow mask perceived as convex can be observed in another video on YouTube (https://www.youtube.com/watch?v=BaofyuCXZ_0).

The two types of observation are as follows:

1. View of the object with parallax movement: The observer looks with one eye at the masks or the landscape, while these objects move to the right or left. Parallax vision implies the optical illusion that objects closer to the observer move faster than objects that are further away. Depending on the perceived speed of movement, one can tell whether an object or part of an object is further or closer to the observer. In this way, an object is perceived as concave or convex.
2. Binocular vision of the object: Binocular vision allows the viewer to recognize the three-dimensionality of the observed object and provides information about its concave or convex perspectival shape (Fig. 5.17).

How did the individuals with schizophrenia and the control group respond to this experiment? Both groups gave the correct answer more than 98% of the time: *Convex* in relation to the convex stimulus, with no significant differences between the two groups of subjects. However, the two groups showed major differences as regards their responses to the *concave* stimuli:

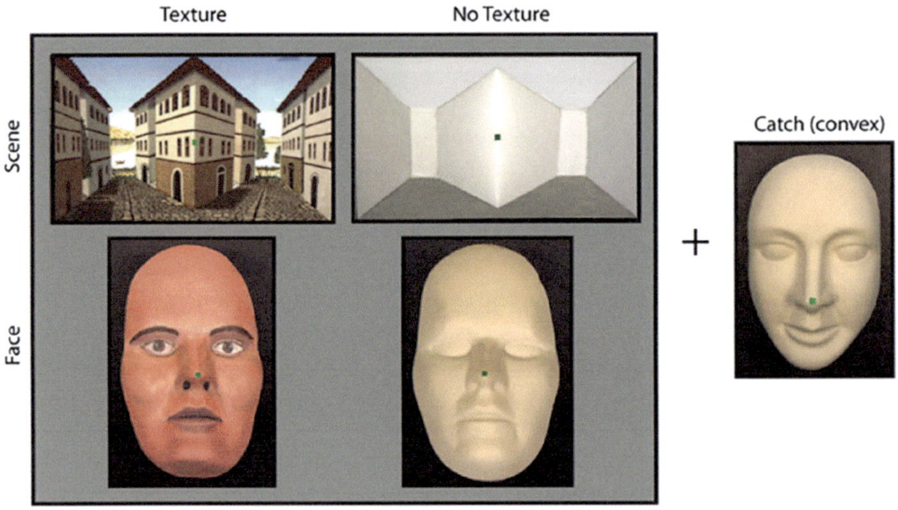

Fig. 5.16 Stimuli for the depth inversion illusions. Subjects observed concave faces and scenes shown with or without misleading painting. Due to the concavity, the green fixation points were further away from the observer than the surrounding regions (cheeks or landscape). A beige face was convex and served as distractor (Keane et al., 2013, p. 507)

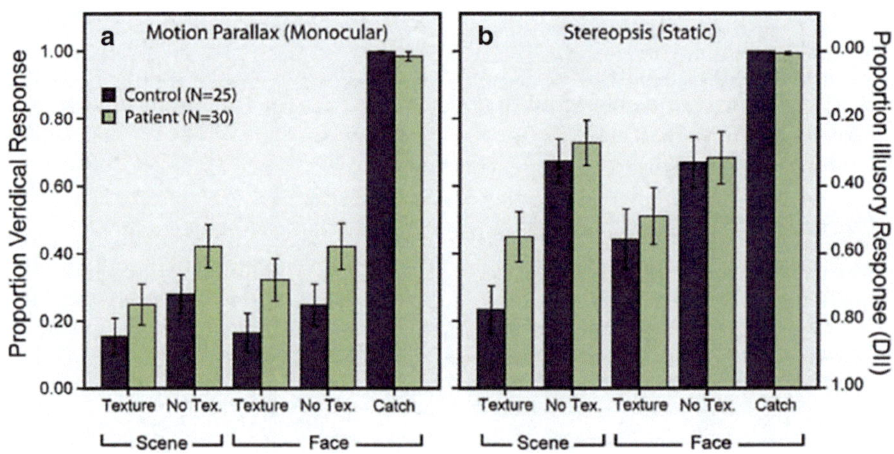

Fig. 5.17 (**a**, **b**) Graph of the results of the stereoscopy test (I). For concave objects, patients gave more truthful responses regardless of object type or viewing condition (Keane et al., 2013, p. 510)

> Patients experienced DIIs less than non-schizophrenic controls and this group difference did not depend on viewing condition (parallax/stereopsis), texture (realistic/blank), or object category (faces/scenes). Notably, the group difference arose when the analyses were restricted only to monocular viewing or only to scenes. For all subjects, performance did not correlate with age, education (mother, father, or self), full-scale IQ, or visual acuity. [...] Patients exhibited less illusion with stereopsis than without, and more illusion with texture than without. (Keane et al., 2013, p. 509 f.)

Three years later, a methodologically identical study was conducted by the same researchers; however, also a group of patients with a bipolar disorder was included (Keane et al., 2016, pp. 485–492).

30 subjects with a bipolar disorder, 30 individuals with schizophrenia, and 25 non-schizophrenic subjects participated in the study. Again, more than 98% of all participants gave correct responses about the convex mask stimulus.

The bipolar group did not respond significantly differently to the depth reversal test than the control group. The only significant difference that emerged in this study concerned the group of individuals with schizophrenia, which confirmed the results of the previous study.

Fig. 5.18c gives an overview of all data collected during the study. Here, the essential difference between the individuals with schizophrenia and the two other groups (bipolar and control group) can be clearly seen.

Further evidence for the validity of these findings is provided by a study on the binocular inversion of concave and convex (Koethe et al., 2009, pp. 195–202). 313 individuals took part in the study: 75 paranoid antipsychotic-naïve individuals with schizophrenia (SZ-N, i.e., never treated with antipsychotics), 74 paranoid individuals with schizophrenia who had been treated with antipsychotics (SZ-T), 22 patients with an initial prodromal state of psychosis (IPS), 35 with a major depressive disorder (MDD), 20 with a bipolar disorder (BD), 6 with Alzheimer's dementia (D), and 81 healthy controls (HC).

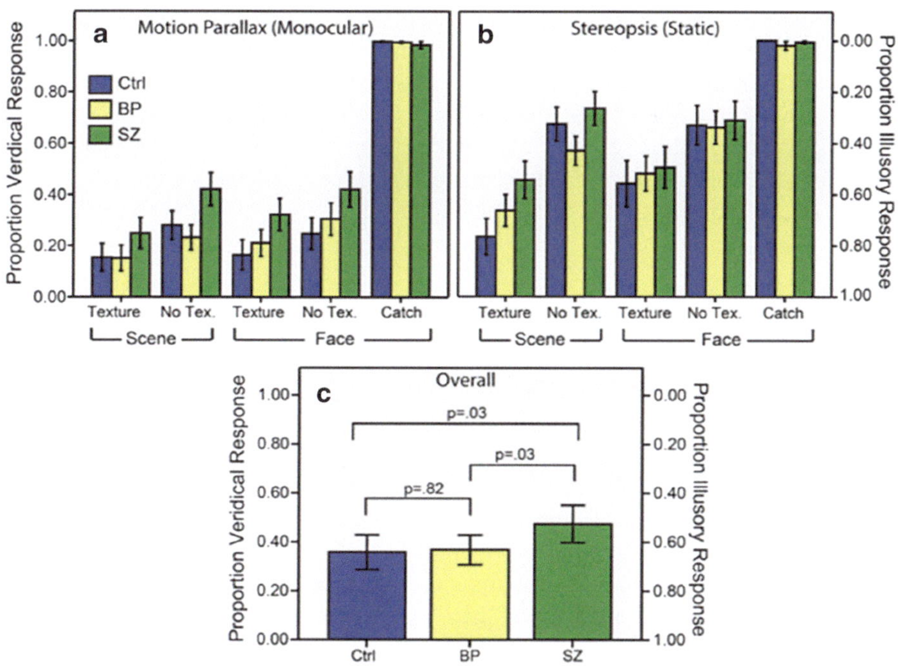

Fig. 5.18 Graph of the results of the stereoscopy test (II) (Keane et al., 2016)

> We investigated the hypothesis that binocular depth inversion illusion (BDII), a visual, 'top-down' driven information process, is impaired in schizophrenia and particularly in its early stages, but neither in non-schizophrenic controls in other major psychiatric illnesses. In accordance with our hypothesis, patients suffering from either initial prodromal state of psychosis (IPS) or from first-episode, antipsychotic-naïve schizophrenia (SZ-N) showed significantly higher scores of the BDII score 'faces' compared to non-schizophrenic controls (HC), indicating that visual processing is already disturbed at this early state of the disease. In accordance with previous studies, BDII scores in short-term antipsychotically treated patients with schizophrenia (SZ-T) were significantly higher than HC. [...] Interestingly, differences between the groups IPS, SZ-N and SZ-T were not statistically different in our study. [...] Our study investigated for the first time disturbances in visual information processing using the BDII not only in schizophrenia spectrum disorders but also in distinct groups of patients suffering depression, bipolar disorder or dementia. For these groups of patients, we found no statistically significant difference compared to non-schizophrenic controls. (Koethe et al., 2009, p. 199 f.)

Many hypotheses have been put forward as to why individuals with schizophrenia are not deceived by the illusion of depth reversal as much as non-schizophrenic individuals or other types of psychiatric patients: One reasonable interpretation of this phenomenon is that individuals with schizophrenia get bogged down with the processing of details of a structure, i.e., in the bottom-up perception phase, and that they do not achieve a whole picture from which they can relationally process the details in a top-down perception. Whatever the neurophysiopathological finding behind this deficit is, from a purely phenomenological point of view one can state that individuals with schizophrenia are impaired in their handling of perspective, three-dimensional vision, visual depth, and the overall coherence of composition. Three-dimensional perspectival vision (however illusory or real it may be) is only possible when the various elements of a composition (both the elements of a face and those of a landscape) are perceived in their mutual relationships. This finding corresponds to the loosening of associations described by Bleuler. When a face is perceived holistically—in the Gestalt-psychological sense—the details that indicate the hollow form are overlooked. Since holistic vision is impaired in schizophrenia, these details continue to be perceived, i.e., the hollow form becomes clearly visible.

5.3.3 Stereoscopy

If it is true that individuals with schizophrenia have problems with three-dimensional or perspectival vision, specific deficits should also be revealed in stereoscopic vision tests. In addition to individuals with schizophrenia, altered spatial depth perception has also been found in subjects with schizotypal personalities (Barbato et al., 2012, pp. 115–132).

In order to see an object stereoscopically at a distance of 3 meters, the brain has to integrate images from both eyes which differ only minimally due to the natural interpupillary distance of approx. 60 mm. The two images are matched, and a three-dimensional image is created from them (Backus et al., 2001, pp. 2054–2068; Nishida et al., 2001, pp. 2259–2263).

The New York research group led by Isaac Schechter (Schechter et al., 2006, pp. 1282–1284) used the graded circles stereo test (Kantrowitz et al., 2009, p. 1089) to investigate the possible differences in stereoscopic perception between two groups of 17 individuals with schizophrenia and 19 non-schizophrenic individuals.

The test consists of nine sets of four circles each (Fig. 5.19). For each set, the observer must choose which of the four circles appears three-dimensional. Each set has an increasing level of difficulty, with the result that the assessment of three-dimensionality becomes more difficult as the task progresses.

The degree of difficulty increases from number 1 to number 9. As can be clearly seen in set 1, the circle appears displaced at the bottom; if this is observed with special polarized glasses and with an intact stereoscopic perception, it appears to protrude out of the plane of the screen. The results of the experiment (Fig. 5.20) confirm the impairment of the perception of three-dimensionality and depth of field in individuals with schizophrenia:

> Stereoacuity for patients on the Graded Circles Stereo Test (mean = 142 arcseconds, median = 100 arcseconds, 95% confidence interval [CI]) was significantly elevated compared with control subjects (mean = 55 arcseconds, median = 40 arcseconds, 95% CI: 40–71; p = 0.006). Furthermore, the percentage of patients with correct stereopsis detection was significantly reduced at 200, 140, 60 and 50 arcseconds compared with control subjects. [...] This study demonstrates that patients with schizophrenia have a marked deficit in binocular depth perception. (Schechter et al., 2006, p. 1283)

The neurophysiological mechanism underlying stereoscopy is still controversial. Most studies assume that individuals with schizophrenia are impaired as regards the magnocellular sensitivity (Coleman et al., 2009, pp. 1108–1116), which is thought to be responsible for stereoscopic vision (Butler et al., 2005, pp. 151–157; Butler et al., 2007, pp. 417–430; Green et al., 1994, pp. 945–951; Keri et al., 2004, pp. 537–542). Other studies, such as those by B. C. Skottun and J. R. Skoyles,

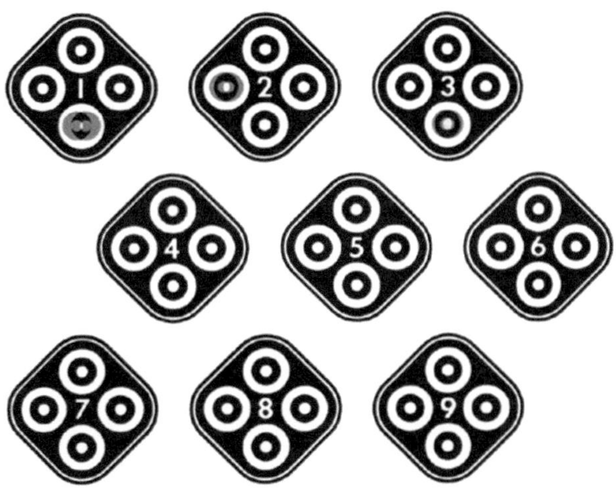

Fig. 5.19 Graded circles stereo test. When viewed with polarized glasses and intact stereoscopy, the circles appear to the viewer as facing forward. In the test series, the degree of difficulty increases progressively (Schechter et al., 2006, p. 1283)

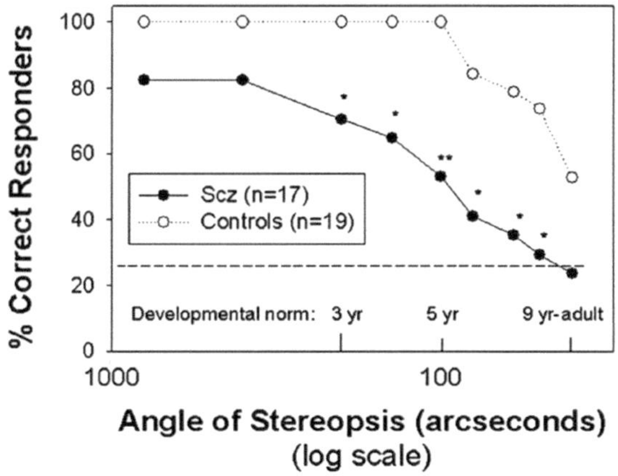

Fig. 5.20 Results of the graded circles stereo test. Comparison in percent of the answers given by the two groups (Schechter et al., 2006, p. 1283)

theorize that stereoscopy is related to parvocellular sensitivity (Skottun & Skoyles, 2009, pp. 697–701).

The presented experiments have clearly shown that spatial perception in schizophrenia cannot result in an overall picture, and consequently, it becomes impossible to develop a holistic perspective.

5.4 Summary

In this chapter, the terms *frame* and *perspective* have been explicated in relation to spatial perception. The frame as a dispositive that guarantees a unified presentation and representation proves to be problematic in individuals with schizophrenia. Their problem apparently consists in integrating visual information into an overall picture or Gestalt, with the result that the uniform perception of space and the constitution of an overall picture are both impaired. However, the frame also plays a central role in relation to social environment, with the result that patients with schizophrenia often do not observe and experience the social environment as a whole.

Perspective, which is correlated with frame, is shown to be impaired in schizophrenic spatial perception. The tests that have analyzed the ability of individuals with schizophrenia to perceive concave and convex shapes as well as their depth and stereoscopic perception indicate a relevant deficit in comparison with non-schizophrenic subjects. Another type of study examining orientation ability has shown a tendency in individuals with schizophrenia to be better at orienting themselves in an egocentric perspective, a perspective experienced idiosyncratically by the subject, than in an allocentric perspective, which is better handled by non-schizophrenic subjects.

Analysis of the Perception of Time

6

6.1 Introduction

This chapter on temporality and phenomenological perception of time by individuals with schizophrenia deals with the philosophical panorama in which clinical observation is embedded: Everything that is linguistically or artistically expressed and spatially experienced takes place in time. Time is the dimension of dimensions; it is the original structure of being and existence (Heidegger, 1927).

The question of time has fascinated philosophers of the Western tradition from the pre-Socratics to the present day. The investigation must be limited directly to the method and the main object of this work: the phenomenological reflections in both philosophy and psychiatry that have created the basic categories necessary for the development of phenomenological psychopathology.

6.2 Philosophical Background

This chapter will elaborate on how the guiding concepts of this book, i.e., how *subjectivity*, *frame*, and *perspective*, emerge from both philosophical and clinical psychiatric analysis.

The key concept which is most useful and appropriate to begin and through which the context of thoughts will unfold is that of *association*. Association forms a crucial concept for Bleuler, in particular, who first characterized schizophrenia as a loosening or loss of associations (Bleuler, 1911; Frith & Johnstone, 2003, p. 30). However, it is also a significant term for the whole of phenomenological philosophy, which, since Husserl, has attempted to describe consciousness in its basic features. In the transition from modernity to postmodernity, subject and reality are strongly reconsidered and experience a deep crisis (Bauman, 1999; Butler, 2002; Chiurazzi, 2007; Giddens, 1990; Jameson, 1989; Lyotard, 1979). Marx teaches that cultural ideas and religious beliefs are a product of economics (Marx, 1867). Freud

P. Parisi, *A Phenomenological Interpretation of Schizophrenia*,
https://doi.org/10.1007/978-3-031-67860-8_6

discovers the invisible dimension of the acting human being, of will and desire, and he questions the lucid rational self-determination of the subject. Finally, Nietzsche represents, as it were, an earthquake in philosophy by reevaluating all the hitherto stable values in which the West had believed since Plato and Paul. Moreover, it was Nietzsche himself who, in Aphorism 125 in *Die fröhliche Wissenschaft* (*The Gay Science*), stated the human, existential, and cultural fragmentation of our time (Nietzsche, 1882, pp. 480–482). In a world in which the rational certainty of thought and the determinism of science had failed, coinciding with the crisis of positivism (Mangoni, 2013), Husserl attempted to create a new foundation for epistemology: His phenomenological method aims at returning to the things themselves, to gain knowledge by explore their basic structures (their *essences*).

Since it is impossible to fully illustrate the scope of Husserl's thinking here (Luft & Wehrle, 2017; Raggiunti, 2007), we will consider Husserl's work that had the greatest influence on the phenomenological reflection on the perception of time: *Zur Phänomenologie des Inneren Zeitbewusstseins* (*On the Phenomenology of Internal Time Consciousness*) (Husserl, 1928). Husserl's reflections aim at analyzing time as an experience lived by consciousness and not through analyzing it purely in the form of objective, quantifiable, or other scientifically measurable data. Consciousness unifies impressions of perception that are experienced discretely in themselves. Husserl gives as an example:

> Thus, for example, a discrete succession can be held together without prejudice to the lack of simultaneity of its members through a bond of consciousness, through a unitary apprehension. That several successive tones yield a melody is possible only in this way, that the succession of psychical processes are united 'forthwith' in a common structure. They are in consciousness one after the other, but they fall within one and the same common act. We do not have the sounds all at once, as it were, and we do not hear the melody by virtue of the circumstance that the earlier tones endure with the last. Rather, the tones build up a successive unity with a common effect, the form of apprehension. (Husserl, 2019, p. 48)

A unified overall picture is the task of a non-schizophrenic consciousness, which can be understood as the embodied synthesis of the three moments of lived temporality, namely, past (retention), present (impression or presentation), and future (protention). The Husserlian view of the lived dimensions of time is literally conceptualized in terms of perspective and is oriented towards subjectivity. Just as spatial perspective organizes objects according to proximity and distance, so does temporal perspective. So that there is perspective, there must also be a frame, an element that gives all perceived things a coherence, that is, a unity. There is a passage in Husserl's work that makes the importance of the frame clear:

> The foreground is nothing without the background; the appearing side is nothing without the non-appearing. It is the same with regard to the unity of time-consciousness—the duration reproduced is the foreground; the classifying intentions make us aware of a background, a temporal background. And in certain ways, this is continued in the constitution of the temporality of the enduring thing itself with its now, before, and after. We have the following analogies: for the spatial thing, the ordering into the surrounding space and the spatial world on the one side, and on the other, the spatial thing itself with its foreground and background. For the temporal thing, we have the ordering into the temporal form and

> the temporal world on the one side, and on the other the temporal thing itself and its changing orientation with regard to the living now. (Husserl, 2019, p. 100)

Husserl's approach is clear and precise. His text offers many examples from everyday life to argue or explain what he intends to demonstrate on a more speculative and theoretical level. The following example, taken from music, a discipline that Husserl particularly valued, is intended to further underline the unity of consciousness:

> Let us now consider the self-evident consciousness of duration and analyze this consciousness itself. If the note C is perceived (and not merely the quality C, but the entire tonal content, which must remain absolutely unaltered) and given as enduring, then the note C is extended over an interval of the immediate temporal field, i.e., another note does not appear in each now but always and continually the same note. That the same note always appears, that there is this continuity of identity, is an internal characteristic of consciousness. The temporal positions are not separated from one another through divisive acts. The unity of perception is here a breachless unity which dispenses with all interrupting internal differences. On the other hand, differences do exist so far as every temporal point is distinct from every other—only distinct, however, not separated. (Husserl, 2019, p. 148)

The representation of the unity of the *inner time consciousness* found much resonance in Europe and thus had consequences in various cultural areas. To give just one example from the world of art: With Cubism, Picasso introduces time, the passing of time, and the inner synthesis of time consciousness into figurative art (Nigro Covre, 2017; Schapiro, 2003). Thus, in *Les Demoiselles d'Avignon* of 1907, the Spanish painter approaches the object from different visual angles that revolve around the depicted object. He breaks down visual perception into its components and then reassembles them, leaving a trail of movement. Furthermore, the theme of stream of consciousness has been used in famous literary works such as *Finnegans Wake* by Joyce (1939), *A la recherche du temps perdu (In Search of Lost Time)* by Proust (1913), or *La coscienza di Zeno (Zeno's Conscience)* by Svevo (1923).

Husserl's reflection, together with earlier reflections by Egger (1881), James (1890), and Bergson (1889, 1896, 1907), created the philosophical preconditions for phenomenological reflection in the clinical and psychiatric field (Cazzullo & Sini, 1984; Fuchs, 2007, 2013, 2017a; Galimberti, 1979; Minkowski et al., 2013; Molaro & Civita, 2012; Roni, 2016; Sini, 2014). It is indeed no coincidence that the meaningful and now classic phenomenological description of time perception in schizophrenia comes from a doctor with an immense philosophical gift, the Bergson disciple Eugène Minkowski; we will return to this idea later.

Before we will deal directly with psychiatric phenomenology, another important author who, a few decades after Husserl, was able to explore and philosophically deepen human perception and epistemology should be mentioned. It is the Frenchman Maurice Merleau-Ponty and his book *Phénoménologie de la perception (Phenomenology of Perception)* (Merleau-Ponty, 1945).

Merleau-Ponty takes up Husserl's phenomenology almost in unison: Some examples he quotes come directly from the German philosopher. In the following section, Merleau-Ponty emphasizes that the body, as a perceiving body, performs a spontaneous synthesis of its being in the world, i.e., in space and time. There is a clear reference here to Husserl's work *Analysen zur passiven Synthese. Aus Vorlesungs- und Forschungsmanukripten 1918–1926* (*Analyses of Passive Synthesis. From Lecture and Research Manuscripts 1918–1926*) (Husserl, 1966, Vol. XI).

> In so far as I have a body through which I act in the world, space and time are not, for me, a collection of adjacent points nor are they a limitless number of relations synthesized by my consciousness, and into which it draws my body. I am not in space and time, nor do I conceive space and time; I belong to them, my body combines with them and includes them. The scope of this inclusion is the measure of that of my existence; but in any case, it can never be all-embracing. The space and time which I inhabit are always in their different ways indeterminate horizons which contain other points of view. The synthesis of both time and space is a task that always has to be performed afresh. (Merleau-Ponty, 2002, p. 187)

Merleau-Ponty introduces terms relevant to our discourse here: The synthesis produced by phenomenological perception is a continuous conquest of perspectives and horizons. The horizon is the ultimate dimension in which all objects of perception find their place. There can be no perspective except from a subject to an object. To better understand the meaning of horizon and phenomenological temporality, it is necessary to first clarify the relationship between subject and object.

> As soon as there is consciousness, and in order that there may be consciousness, there must be something to be conscious of, an intentional object, and consciousness can move towards this object only to the extent that it 'derealizes' itself and throws itself into it, only if it is wholly in this reference to… something, only if it is a pure meaning-giving act. If a being is consciousness, he must be nothing but a network of intentions. If he ceases to be definable in terms of the act of sense-giving, he relapses into the condition of a thing, the thing being precisely what does not know, what slumbers in absolute ignorance of itself and the world, what consequently is not a true 'self,' i.e., a 'for-itself,' and has only a spatio-temporal form of individuation, existence in itself. (Merleau-Ponty, 2002, p. 165)

Subjectivity gains its perspective and its horizon and integrates the various dimensions of lived space-time in the present. The synthesis of perspectives is not given as an object among objects but is the fruit of subjectivity and constitutes its activity. According to Merleau-Ponty, subject and perspective can also be placed in one. In the following section, we read about the importance of time for the synthetic perception not only of temporality but also of the subjective and objective world as a whole:

> Through my perceptual field, with its spatial horizons, I am present to my surrounding, I co-exist with all the other landscapes which stretch out beyond it, and all these perspectives together form a single temporal wave, one of the world's instants. Through my perceptual field with its temporal horizons, I am present to my present, to all the preceding past and to a future. And, at the same time, this ubiquity is not strictly real, but is clearly only intentional. (Merleau-Ponty, 2002, p. 411)

This passage, which summarises the importance of temporal perspective for the perceiving subject, is found towards the end of Merleau-Ponty's book in which he describes the connection between time and the subject:

> This amounts to saying that each present reasserts the presence of the whole past which it supplants, and anticipates that of all that is to come, and that by definition the present is not shut up within itself but transcends itself towards a future and a past. [...] The past, therefore, is not past, nor the future future. It exists only when a subjectivity is there to disrupt the plenitude of being in itself, to adumbrate a perspective, and introduce non-being into it. A past and a future spring forth when I reach out towards them. I am not, for myself, at this very moment, I am also at this morning or at the night which will soon be here, and though my present is, if we wish so to consider it, this instant, it is equally this day, this year or my whole life. [...] We must understand time as the subject and the subject as time. (Merleau-Ponty, 2002, pp. 513–515)

If for Maurice Merleau-Ponty time is the subject and the subject time, then it can be concluded that subject and time are ultimately perspective. More precisely, the subject is a bundle of perspectives. The plural is necessary in this case because time and subject transcend the perspectives continuously. This point is fundamental because the subject is always producing new horizons and syntheses from perspectives. This point will be developed further in the conclusion.

6.3 Temporality of Frame and Perspective in Schizophrenia

From the hermeneutic-textual analysis of these two key works of twentieth-century phenomenological thought, significant elements have emerged that shed new light on our work. If it is true that the subject is time and perspective, as has been said so far, at least in its non-schizophrenic state, then we see an altered synthesis of temporality in psychiatric pathologies, especially in the case of schizophrenia, where subjectivity is clearly impaired.

As already mentioned, the author who most influenced the debate on the phenomenological interpretation of temporality in schizophrenia was Minkowski (1927, 1933). Minkowski takes up the conceptual categories developed by Husserl and Bergson, emphasizing the centrality of the concepts of perspective and horizon. The subject is conceived as a center that is able to condense past and present experiences in itself and then to open itself to the future with the *élan vital* defined by Bergson.

This *élan* is the perspective on the future. To speak about temporality without taking spatiality into account is impossible, and Minkowski knows this very well. In dealing with the dimension of the future, Minkowski suggests that:

> We look at the future and we see it in a broad and majestic perspective stretching out to lose itself in the distance. This majesty approaches the mysterious. But this mystery is as indispensable to our spiritual life as pure air is to our respiration. It makes of the future a reservoir of eternal and inexhaustible forces without which we could not continue to live. See how far we are from the idea of the uniform succession of events and the straight line which was to represent time in this succession! A spatial image is much too weak to express the power of the future, which has extension, grandeur, power in it. (Minkowski, 1970, p. 117)

Here, Minkowski considers different metaphors. The spatial metaphor seems to fall short for him. Yet he attempts to introduce a further spatial image.

> An image comes involuntarily to the mind—that of horizon, where, when our gaze turns toward infinity, the sky blends with the earth. That is a spatial and metaphorical image, someone will say. This occurred to me also, yet I was not convinced. Rather, the image of the horizon and the vision of the future fit very well together. They blend together, and when we want to distinguish them, it becomes impossible to say which of them is the more original and which borrows its elements from the other. [...] Moreover, when we open our eyes and when we say that we look in front of us, is this 'in front' a mere convention, a name agreed to in common, or on the contrary doesn't it have something absolute in it? Isn't it an 'in front' or a 'before' which is real and irreversible, a perspective toward which we are completely prepared to rush? And doesn't this 'before' point to time and the future rather than to space? What passionate questions, which, from the manner in which they are posed, seem to indicate the response they require. (Minkowski, 1970, p. 117)

In bringing together the concepts of time and space, this passage provides us with the possibility of imagining not only time and space as separate dimensions of experience but as a unified time-spatial dimension of the experiencing human being:

> If I do not give this response immediately, perhaps I will be able to give it later, perhaps I have even given it already. The idea of spatiotemporal solidarity increasingly comes to mind. We see at the same time the problem of lived space appear, waiting in the distance, space which will not dissect or immobilize time in modeling it in its own way. On the contrary, time bears it within itself and vivifies it to the highest degree in filling it with all that is mobile and dynamic in it. In any case, when with regard to time we speak of extension, or perspective, or of horizon, that seems very far from a simple metaphor. On the contrary, we seem to be concerned with the essential characteristics of the future, which belong to it to the same degree as the corresponding givens of a spatial kind. (Minkowski, 1970, p. 117)

This quotation is important because it merges the perception of space that has been described in the previous chapter and the perception of time that is described in this chapter. This opens up a way of comprehending the importance of the space-time perspective in human life. Moreover, it is precisely this way of understanding lived time that individuals with schizophrenia lack, namely, the drive towards the future. According to Minkowski, the difference between healthy, non-schizophrenic individuals and individuals with schizophrenia is that the lack of vital energy can affect the life of each of us, diminishing any enthusiasm for the future. In non-schizophrenic individuals, these states are merely transitory and are usually overcome. An individual with schizophrenia, on the other hand, lives constantly in an existential state in which the future can no longer be thought about. Consequently, the days flow like a repetitive river, without the anticipation and sense of the opportunities brought by each new day (cf. Minkowski, 1933, Volume II). In the course of the treatise, Minkowski reports in detail (also on the basis of earlier studies by Franz Fischer) clinical cases in which patients with schizophrenia lose their *élan* towards their future. Accordingly, the past also seems to lose depth, and the only truly perceived temporal dimension remains that of the present:

> Attacked in his vital dynamism, the schizophrenic not only seems completely immobilized in himself but seems as if deprived of the necessary organ to assimilate anything dynamic, and he lives outside himself. [...] Everything around me is immobile. Things appear isolated, each one in itself, without suggesting anything. Certain things which ought to evoke

> memory, evoke an immense number of thoughts, present a picture, remain isolated. [...] The creative power in me is abolished. I see the future as a repetition of the past. (Minkowski, 1970, p. 117)

That in individuals with schizophrenia the perception of time is reduced to the present and loses historical depth, and future perspective has been reported by several authors, including the aforementioned Fischer (1929), Fischer (1930a, 1930b), Schilder (1942, p. 217), Borgna (1995, pp. 108–109), Muscelli and Stanghellini (2012), and De Martino (1977, pp. 133–140).

Anticipating Blankenburg's grand psychiatric conception, Minkowski speaks of the "loss of vital contact with reality." An individual with schizophrenia lacks association, both the association between spatial elements and temporal points, on the one hand, and the association of himself with the world of life, on the other hand.

Klaus Conrad pointed out something similar when he described the phases of trema, delusional mood, and delusional perception. The schizophrenia patient experiences a delusional mood in which the ego slowly seems to lose control over reality and the passage of time (Conrad, 1959, pp. 63–149).

The Japanese psychopathologist Bin Kimura sees the individual with schizophrenia as suspended in time by defining the schizophrenia patient's perception of temporality as *ante festum* (Kimura, 1992). According to Kimura, individuals with schizophrenia live in an imaginary future. This dimension of time is disconnected from the classical division of time into past, present, and future. We can therefore confirm that the *ante festum* time dimension that Kimura speaks of is always a punctual, floating, non-relational time. One can only have an awareness of the future once one is cognizant of the present. The *ante festum experience* seems to be a future that falls instead into the present, a future that is present in every moment of the schizophrenic's life, and a future that is a present in the guise of a future. The psychiatrist and phenomenologist Stanghellini (2006) also appears to support this thesis in his commentary on Kimura:

> Persons with schizophrenia were also described as living in an elusive, eternal and pregnant 'now' called the ante festum, in which what is most important is always about to happen. Especially in early schizophrenia, time is suspended: it is a paradoxical mixture of immobility and protention, a knot of stillness and incipient moment. Temporal fragmentation has been considered as a generative disturbance in schizophrenia. Major schizophrenic symptoms (e.g., thought insertion, hallucinations or passivity experiences) have been regarded as manifesting a disturbance of the constitutive synthesis of time consciousness. (Stanghellini et al., 2016, p. 46)

Minkowski speaks of a loss of contact with reality, which points not only to the problematic relationship between subject and world but also and above all between subject and lived time. Blankenburg (1991) engages himself in an extensive analysis of temporality in schizophrenia. His considerations are fundamental for the further development of our thesis. The concept of frame is explicitly introduced in relation to time. This concept emerges here in all its significance. The terms *subjectivity*, *frame*, and *perspective* are thus used in different interpretations by the great psychiatrists of the twentieth century. Blankenburg presents the clinical case of Ms. A.:

> A. complained that every morning 'everything always seems quite different' to her. When asked what was different, she could not give a proper answer; rather out of a certain embarrassment she said: 'life, duties, being human...,' these words seeming to her insufficient for what she meant. It was not the individual things that had changed, she could remember all the details of the previous day well, but the frame within which everything stood was different.

Blankenburg interpreted:

> She obviously suffered from a lack of continuity backwards, but of a particular kind. It was not a matter of the relationship to the objectively comprehensible passage of time, for instance mnestic disturbances in the narrower sense, and yet the relationship to the past was altered in a profound way. [...] The existence lacks the wherefrom. This wherefrom is not itself localizable within a quantitatively understood dimension of time but is qualitative in nature. [...] The lack of a backward reference thus denies her the prospective progression forwards.

Blankenburg quotes the patient:

> It is so hard for me to stay in reality. Every day I have to start again, all over again!

He interprets her with reference to the concept of the frame:

> Thus, it is clear enough that it is precisely this 'as yesterday so today and tomorrow' that is missing. And A. knows that this also endangers her remaining in reality, i.e., the reality of everyday existence. What she cannot connect with are not the details of the previous day but 'rather the principles', the 'framework' in which everything takes place. She then feels herself each time as anew, as if she were in another world, without knowing how to describe this other world in a positive way. It is not a delusional world. And yet, through this alteration of the temporalization, she is transferred out of the world we share into a world of her own, however little it seems to be filled with concrete contents of her own world. The continuity-building moment of Dasein, "that it, living into its days, extends 'temporally' in the succession of its days" (Heidegger) is affected, and that alone already means a modification of the worldliness of the world. (Blankenburg, 1991, pp. 113–115. Source in German)

So far, each author has added an important piece of the mosaic to our developing picture. However, although the concepts of perspective and frame have been treated in depth so far, it remains to be clarified how schizophrenic subjectivity relates to its fragmentary and momentary experience of time. As has already been noted elsewhere (Fuchs, 2007, p. 231), Husserl described the phenomenology of retention in greater detail than that of protention. According to Minkowski's interpretation, we gain stability from our orientation towards the future.

When the temporal perspective in which our thoughts, our will, our desires, our plans unfold fails, what is left? How can the intentional arc that Maurice Merleau-Ponty speaks of be reconsidered in the impaired perception of temporality in schizophrenia? This question was answered by the phenomenological reflection of the philosopher and psychiatrist Thomas Fuchs. In an article on this topic, Fuchs offers with precision the graphic visualization of protention (Figs. 6.1, 6.2, and 6.3) as

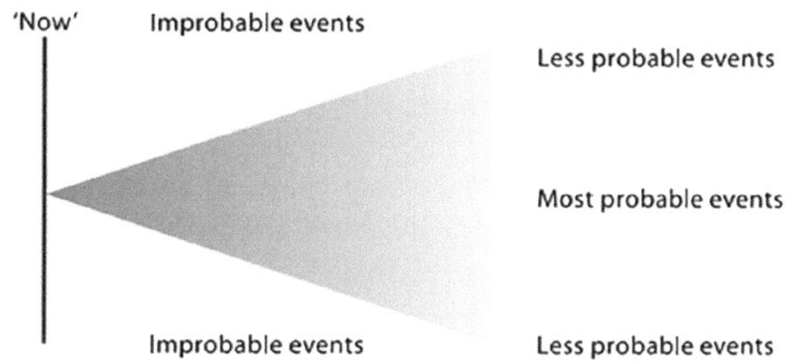

Fig. 6.1 Protentional function (Fuchs, 2007, p. 231)

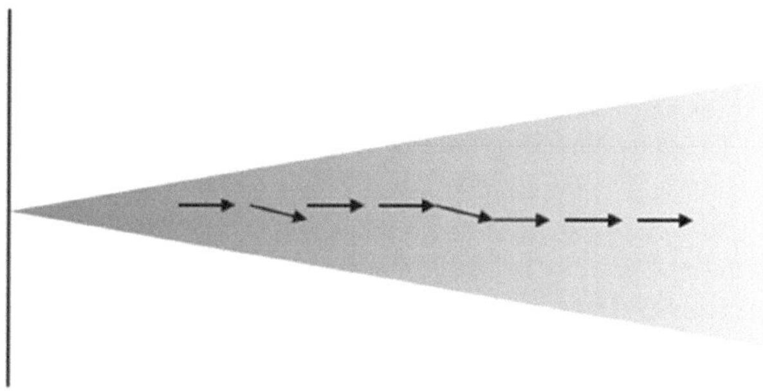

Fig. 6.2 Focused protention (e.g., during focused thinking and speaking) (Fuchs, 2007, p. 231)

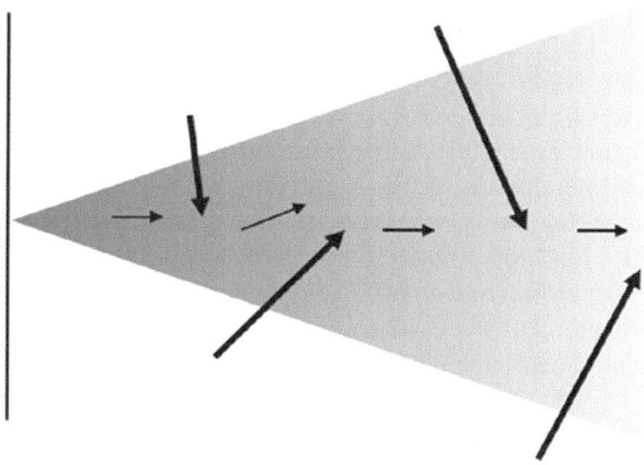

Fig. 6.3 Fragmented protention in schizophrenia (Fuchs, 2007, p. 234)

experienced by the non-schizophrenic subject and as experienced by the subject with schizophrenia (Fuchs, 2007, p. 231 ff.).

According to Fuchs, in non-schizophrenic individuals, protention opens up into a probability cone that tends to remain narrow when it is strongly focused on a purpose and intention to be pursued. Protention is defined as the anticipation of internal or external events, such as playing a musical instrument, moving an object, and forming a thought or speech (Fuchs, 2007, p. 213). The non-schizophrenic subject is thereby thought of as a center capable of organizing the means to achieve an end. The German adjective *zielorientiert* is not easy to translate into other languages and shows its descriptive and explanatory effect: A *goal-oriented* person is basically *oriented towards a goal*. In individuals with schizophrenia, on the other hand, whose subjectivity is impaired, there is an expansion of the probability cone indicating the lack of effectiveness of the subject's protentional, goal-oriented capacity.

The intentional arc is fragmented allowing disturbing ideas or intrusions to invade the flow of thought or speech. The schizophrenic proves unable to focus attention on the outside world and on drawing up a plan for the future. The relationship between subject and object is damaged, leaving the subject isolated in his own dimension, his own time, and his own world. Fuchs describes this as follows:

> Schizophrenic experience of reference, persecution and control may thus be explained by an 'inversion of intentionality': with the paralysis of the patient's own intentional activity, the direction of his mental acts is reversed and turned against him, as if coming from the outside. Instead of actively perceiving, thinking and acting, he is being perceived, related to, thought of and acted upon by others. (Fuchs, 2007, p. 234)

The schema proposed by Fuchs is extremely relevant to the subject-frame-perspective theory. Revised according to this theory, it then presents itself as follows:

Indeed, the schema for the protentional arc outlined by Merleau-Ponty and Fuchs can be extended. The relationship between subject and object presupposes both a perspective and a frame. More precisely, the frame is the precondition for perspectival vision, i.e., here for the protention described by phenomenology. The four elements *subject*, *frame*, *perspective*, and *object* can now be assigned to each other in a summarizing schema (Fig. 6.4). The arrow shows the tension of the subject towards the object at which the intentional arc is directed. The probability cone that Fuchs speaks of corresponds to the left-hand half of the schema. To be intentionally focused on an object, moreover, is to understand what must remain inside and what must remain outside the frame of meaning. The frame separates what is relevant to the protention from what is irrelevant. Only in this way does the object become the true vanishing point of the subject's intentional perspective. And it is precisely this ability to distinguish that is more or less impaired in individuals with schizophrenia, depending on the case.

In the schema presented above, all the so far discussed terms were put into relation: *Subject*, *object*, *perspective*, and *frame* together form a general model of human experience. Moreover, if the perspective on the object is lost in schizophrenia, if the conceptual, hermeneutic, and symbolic frame is lost, then

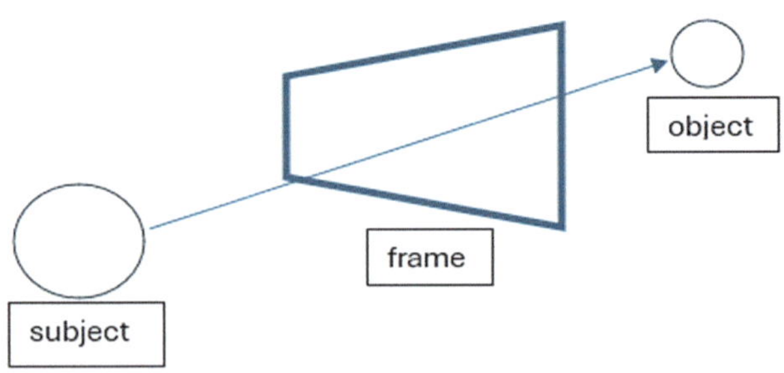

Fig. 6.4 Schema of the relationship between the subject and the object according to the subject-frame-perspective theory (own figure)

non-schizophrenic relational subjectivity is also lost. The reversal of the subject's intentionality on itself, the transition from non-schizophrenic subjectivity to pathological Subjectivation, means the breaking of the connection between the ego (the ontological dimension of the subject) and the self (the objectified representation of the subject), between the ego and the world.

When Thomas Fuchs deals with authors interested in the change of the self in schizophrenia, he offers a classification of the diverse aspects in which the ego of the schizophrenic proves to be impaired and fragmented, as follows: The ego loses (1) reference and stability for itself, (2) the relationship to the environment, and (3) the social or intersubjective relationship (Fuchs, 2012). To these pre-reflexive aspects are added the disturbances of the ego's reflexivity, whereby everything becomes doubtful, uncertain, threatening, and unstable for the ego. This goes so far that some patients can no longer recognize the relationship between themselves and their image reflected in the mirror. Others are unable to integrate time into their ego continuity and therefore cannot experience themselves in their own temporal continuity. The ego breaks down, becomes alien, and then becomes a thing among various other things. It is no longer able to experience itself from its central position.

Both the small gestures of daily life and behavior in society become problematic: They lose their immediacy, spontaneity, and naturalness. Everything that is normally familiar now becomes foreign, distant, new, and confusing. Individuals with schizophrenia can be confronted with the same object in a new way at any moment. Therefore, they lack reliability and trust in reality, in the regularity of the familiar and the habitual. In the German language, *bewohnen* (to inhabit) and *Gewohnheit* (habit), like the Italian words *abitare* and *abitudine*, come from the same root; there is an immanent relationship between these two terms: Individuals with schizophrenia do not live in or inhabit the reality and cannot get used to reality. They live in a suspended time of endless search for their own identity and for the world.

When the continuity of the self is missing, when one loses that centrality from which one can observe with confidence and stability the world offered to the gaze, then one is no longer able to freely choose and compose oneself and one's perspectives. As one of Fuchs' patients puts it:

> Then something strange happens. My consciousness (of myself, of my father, of space, of the physical reality around us) becomes blurred all at once. [...] I think I am dissolving. I feel [...] like a sandcastle with all its sand slipping away into the receding surf. [...] Consciousness is gradually losing its coherence. The center gives way. The center no longer holds. The 'I' becomes a veil, and the fixed center from which one experiences reality breaks down... There is no longer a stable standpoint from which to look out, to take things in, to assess what is happening. No core holds things together anymore or forms the lens through which we otherwise see the world. (Fuchs, 2012, p. 887; source in German)

This patient's account is relevant because it can be read as a summary interpretation of various aspects and components of this work. The subject is the foundation of any play of frames and perspectives; it is the "standpoint" towards which perspectives are centered and frames are set; it is the "core" that "holds things together."

The subject is the "center" that makes the perception of the world, of lived time, of lived space, of everyday experience, and of life coherent.

If the ego does not immediately recognize the self as its own, it cannot recognize the other as an alterity either. Thus, not having one's own perspective means not being able to adopt the perspective of others either. The world of the schizophrenic is a self-referential world, a one-dimensional world in which the self-evidence of real life has been lost.

Fuchs (2012) summarizes the elements that characterize schizophrenia phenomenologically and provides a summary interpretation of this mental disorder. The non-schizophrenic subject learns to act under its own perspective, to adopt the perspectives of others, and to change perspectives in early childhood.

> One must be able to integrate the egocentric and the allocentric perspective without losing one's own bodily center. To put it pointedly, every perspective-taking already implies a potential loss of the self, which, however, is dissolved *in statu nascendi*. Acquiring this flexibility and security of perspective-taking is a decisive step in child development in the 2nd and 3rd year of life. It thus acquires the 'eccentric position' (Plessner, 1975) that allows the primary, lived body-centred perspective and the secondary, decentered perspective to exist in tension with each other and at the same time integrate them. (Fuchs, 2012, p. 897; source in German)

Plessner describes this ability to change perspectives as the ability of people to adopt "eccentric positions." The subject's natural ability to change perspectives is severely impaired in schizophrenia. Fuchs picks up on this and takes it further:

> It is now this dialectical tension of eccentric positionality that the schizophrenia patient can no longer maintain in the encounter with others. Since his anchoring in the bodily center is lost, the two perspectives are no longer integrated, but rather confounded. Thus the patients get into a disembodied, imaginary and delusional perspective that is directed at themselves from outside or from the others. Everyone seems to know about them, everything seems to relate to them, because they are no longer aware of themselves but only see themselves from the outside—lost, as it were, on an eccentric orbit. Precisely because they lose their bodily centre, they become the supposed center of others' gazes and intentions. The 'short-circuit' of the two perspectives can also lead to the delusion of the expansion of thoughts: All of the patient's thoughts seem to be already known to the others because there is no longer any difference between his own consciousness and that of the others. (Fuchs, 2012, p. 897; source in German)

This last passage touches on the three key elements of this book: (1) the impaired subject, whose ontologically impaired subjectivity will be discussed in more detail in the following conclusion; (2) perspective, as the lived body-centered capacity of the subject to acquire its own and others' standpoint or point of view; and (3) frame, as an element of the human capacity for differentiation and as a guarantee of comprehension. Non-schizophrenic persons can immediately recognize themselves as a singular and individual center, in their own identity and subjectivity, although it is in the world and related to all things in the world.

6.4 Summary

The inability to understand the perspective of the other, as we have already seen in the previous chapters, manifests itself as an impaired ability to understand ironic expressions or non-lexicalized metaphors or the facial expressions and proxemics of the body language of the interlocutor. A healthy and natural social life and normal and everyday interactions with others require dealing not only with perspectives but also with frames. Understanding situational, cultural, and social frames is essential for lively and intersubjective interaction. The importance of perspectives and frames for the living subject concerns not only the perception of space and time, as basic dimensions of human perception and experience, but also the subjectivity of the human being, as an inescapable basic dimension and prerequisite of the ego. In this book, the *center* that according to Fuchs is lost to the patient is referred to as the subjectivity of the ego, which is considered the essential core of the person and the person's abilities. When this center can no longer play a secure, fixed, and central role, when it is no longer the fulcrum for the lively play of perspective and the framing, then subjectivity manifests itself as severely impaired. It is precisely this impairment of subjectivity that characterizes schizophrenia as a condition, and it is given the psychopathological name of *Subjectivation*. This theme is discussed in the following conclusion *in extenso*.

Conclusion: Subjectivation, Frame, and Perspective

7

7.1 Frame and Perspective

The present treatise is entirely supported by two concepts: perspective and frame. In each chapter, they play a central role as *condensation nuclei* around which thoughts, reflections, experiments, observations, but also questions have aggregated.

The frame is the dispositive of the human ability to differentiate and the guarantee of the unity of the imagination. It plays a central role in understanding metaphors, irony, and the coherence of a linguistic text. It is also crucial for the analysis of artistic works and drawings. Therefore, it is a central consideration in our analysis of artistic works made by patients with schizophrenia. The concept of frame also proves to be a viable term to describe the human capacity for holistic vision, be it of a face, a drawing, or a surrounding space.

Perspective is the dispositive of the subject's orientation in time, space, and its *being-in-the-world*. Perspective is our way of mapping out time, desires, and plans for the future, of remembering personal and social things from the past. It enables the play of interactions between different actors, and it enables us to explain social communication processes: Understanding irony is a vivid example. Comprehending the other's perspective also means understanding nonverbal language such as gestures, facial expressions, and proxemics. Perspective is the way we observe the reality in which we are immersed and which surrounds us. The concept of perspective is central to our work, for example, in describing drawings. It can be used to show what is special about drawings of schizophrenia patients: A unified perspective is often absent; the drawings are sometimes disorganized, insecure, or distorted with regard to perspective.

Perspective and frame are therefore two keywords that effectively describe the clinic of schizophrenia: impairments in the perception of spatiality and temporality, impairment of speech and thought, artistic expression, and interpersonal communication.

P. Parisi, *A Phenomenological Interpretation of Schizophrenia*,
https://doi.org/10.1007/978-3-031-67860-8_7

The innovation of this work is in showing that with the concepts of perspective and frame it is possible to see the many different clinical manifestations of schizophrenia under a unified interpretive paradigm. The concepts of perspective and frame make it possible to approach very different symptomatologies in a conceptually unified way. The parallelism emerging in the different impairments is astounding. The two aforementioned concepts allow for a holistic interpretation of the diverse studies that are methodologically and thematically far apart. In a sense, perspective and frame can thus serve as a polestar that can also guide clinicians in their daily work, or in another metaphor: Perspective and frame are the theoretical *vade mecum* that should always be at hand.

The subject's *being-in-the-world* is constituted by perspectives and frames. Although the concept of subjectivity has been developed to a lesser extent in this work than the concepts of perspective and frame, that concept is inescapably presupposed. Schizophrenia is the psychiatric disorder in which the subjectivity of the person is most impaired. Schizophrenia is the disorder of the *I*. The *I* is the fulcrum around which perspectives and frames are flexibly organized, from the small scale of everyday life to the large plans of life. Living a non-schizophrenic life means being able to build, develop, negotiate, relate and integrate perspectives and frames afresh.

For this reason, the underlying concept of subjectivity must now be made systematically explained.

7.2 Subjectivity

Subjectivity is both the transcendental and the embodied dimension of the subject. It is the *non-imaginable*, *the non-objectifiable*, and the *self-givenness* that cannot be objectified.

Phenomenological thinking about subjectivity is essential both for understanding the basic structure of the subject and for understanding schizophrenia as a disorder of the ego.

Thinking about the subject phenomenologically means thinking about it in its constitutive dimension, both intersubjectively and intrasubjectively.

In the phenomenological analysis of the subject, linguistic considerations are crucial because it is through language that we are able to produce the basic categories of thought for the foundation of any science. Thinking about language means thinking about both the possibilities and the limitations of language itself. We therefore reflect on subjectivity starting from the analysis of the subject in language. We note that only in language do human beings as speakers have the possibility of presenting themselves as a subject, as an *ego*.

Every language knows the grammatical category *subject*. There is no language without personal pronouns, even if these may sometimes not be made explicit or are only implied, for moral, social, or situational reasons (Benveniste, 1966, p. 114). The personal pronoun *I* refers to the individual speech act in which it is pronounced and with which it designates the speaker. It always comes into play when the speaker explicitly adopts the first-person perspective. However, when we talk about *the self*, we have to hypostasize it for grammatical reasons. This hypostasizing is misleading insofar as we thereby objectify the *I*. When we talk about the *I*, we have to use the substantivized pronoun, which is imposed on us by the language. The noun substantive *the self* is, however, something quite different from the first person singular pronoun *I*. To think of the *I* under the linguistic category of the noun is to treat it as one thing among others, but we know that this would be a mistake.

When *I* (as a person placed in a certain cultural, social and existential context) think of *myself*, I have to think of myself objectified, as an object. Any use of a pronoun or a substantive form (*the self*) would imply hypostasis, while the speaker is and remains transcendent towards it. Let us consider the following sentences:

X: I am observing myself.

The subject of the sentence is *I*, the verb is *observe*, and the object is *myself*. Anyone who listens to this sentence knows that person X is observing himself or herself, but also notices that the subject, the observing *I*, is something other than the observed object, the *myself*, although *myself* refers to the subject itself. Languages distinguish the pronouns *I* and *myself*, for example, in Italian:

X: Io mi osservo. (I am observing myself.)

X: Io mi piaccio. (I like myself.)

Even here, where nouns are not declined, the forms of the accusative pronouns referring to objects are clearly different from the nominative pronouns referring to the subject. Therefore, the subject cannot reflect upon itself (as subject) linguistically:

X: I think of *I*.

This sentence is grammatically incorrect and therefore nonsensical. I cannot speak about *I*, only about *myself*. However, the grammatical illogicality that appears again and again in different languages concerns not only the linguistic but also the conceptual limit of reflexive thinking.

The personal pronoun *I* has a priority value over the other pronouns. However, there is an *I* only in relation and in contrast to a *you*. Without the pronoun *you*, there would be no pronoun *I* and vice versa. The pronoun of the third person singular is more complex because it denotes the subject who is absent or not directly involved in the dialogue between *I* and *you*.

This is an important point: The pronoun *I* exists when there is a correlative *you*, which means that these pronouns only exist through their interdependence. This is why dialogue is the basic form of language and thought. In Italian, even when one is speaking alone, one speaks *tra sé e sé*, i.e., with oneself and oneself; thus, there is a dialogue between those designated by different pronouns, i.e., between *I* and *myself*. The monologue is an inner dialogue. The French linguist Émile Benveniste notes that in Arabic the first person (*I*) is *al-mutakallimu* (the one who speaks), the second person (*you*) is *al-muhātabu* (the one addressed), and the third person (*he, she, it*) is *al-yā'ibu* (the one who is absent) (Benveniste, 1966, p. 130). These terms indicate the disparity between persons, especially between the third person and the first and second persons. Benveniste notes: "*Interiority and transcendence* are properties of the 'I'" (Benveniste, 1966, p. 135). Sentences about a third person follow a different pattern. To better understand this qualitative difference, let us consider the following sentences:

X: I swear.

X: Y swears.

The two sentences are uttered by the same person, person X. However, the first sentence has a fundamentally different value than the second sentence. The first sentence, in the first person, identifies the utterance with the act itself: The person who says "I swear" thereby performs both the speech act and the act of swearing. Thus, while the first sentence represents a commitment, the second sentence is only a description (Benveniste, 1966, p. 130; Austin, 1962a)

A fundamental principle is: *I* is always and infinitely more than I think I am and more than I can say I am. *I* is the pronoun that indicates the *self-givenness* of the subject's subjectivity. Subjectivity is the unthinkable of the subject; it is the mystery on which every attempt of a formal objectification of thought fails. Subjectivity is the transcendental dimension of the *I*, not a thing among things, but the center of representing oneself.

The *I* organizes the world according to its presence in the world. All languages have some classes of pronouns that depend directly on the personal perspective of the speaker. These are local, temporal, illocutionary, imaginative, and situational deictics: e.g., *this*, *that*, *there*, *now*, *today*, *yesterday*, *tomorrow*, *near*, or *far* only make sense originating from the speaking subject.

The deictics offer a way of establishing a relationship between subject and world. The past and the future are only conceivable starting from a present that is the time in which one speaks. Benveniste brings into play the concept of subjectivity as the basis of perspective:

> The conclusion—surprising at first glance, but in deep accord with the real nature of language—is that the only tense inherent in language is the axial present of discourse, and that this present is implicit. It determines two other temporal references, which must obligatory made explicit. These, in turn, expose the present as the dividing line between that which is no longer and that which is not yet present. These two references do not refer to time, but to views of time, projected backward and forward from the present point. This appears to be the fundamental experience of time, to which all languages bear witness after their fashion. (Benveniste, 1965a, p. 8 f.)

Subjectivity sets temporal perspectives in speech and correlates events to each other in this temporal perspective. The temporal relationships between events have meaning when they relate to the *I* of the speaker.

Subjectivity also sets spatial perspectives in speech and assigns objects to each other in this spatial perspective.

An entity is called near or far only because of the relationship it has to the *I*.

Apart from the principle, which conceives the subject as the transcendental center of deictic experience, there is another principle: Subjectivity grounds dialogical speech and produces time and space in a perspectival manner in relation to the *I*.

In the following, the dimensions of the *I* will be presented in more detail.

The Italian language opens up the possibility of an essential differentiation here. To interrogate the wisdom of language is to apply a phenomenological method. Anchoring this analysis of the *self* in a linguistic analysis is of enormous value. In Italian, *face* is expressed in three different ways: *volto*, *faccia*, and *viso*. In everyday language, these three words are used almost synonymously. However, there is a difference in meaning between these terms. The following differentiation will serve as the starting point for the following phenomenological reflection on the *self*:

1. *Volto* corresponds to the deep and unrecognizable dimension of the person. It corresponds to the *self-givenness* of subjectivity. *Volto* is the innermost part of the human being, what scholasticism and Rhenish-Flemish mysticism called *συνδήρησις* or *vünkelin*, the spark of the soul—Albertus Magnus, Hugo of Strasbourg, Meister Eckhart (De Libera, 1984, p. 193). *Volto* is not only a noun but also the past participle of the verb *volgere*. By definition, *volto* is always "the face turned towards others": It does not open itself, it does not enter into relationship, but it is the basis of every possibility of relationship.
2. *Faccia*: The visible dimension of the person, what the *I* shows to the other. The word *faccia* occurs in many idioms that express relationality in a social context, for instance, *metterci la faccia* (to stand up for it, to stand up for it publicly), *essere sfacciato* (to be insolent), *giocarsi la faccia* (to squander one's reputation, one's credibility], *perdere la faccia* (to lose one's face), *salvare la faccia* (to save one's face), and *avere la faccia tosta di fare qualcosa* (to have the courage to do something). As to the word *facciata* (façade), it is the surface with which a building presents itself to the observer from the outside without revealing anything about the interior. A beautiful façade can hide a dilapidated palace, or a dilapidated façade can hide a beautiful palace. The *faccia*, like the façade, is what individuals reveal about themselves and allows them to enter the social, relational, and intersubjective context.
3. *Viso*: The dimension of the person in the imagination of the other who looks at the person. The expression *viso* concerns the category of intersubjectivity present in *faccia*; however, the perspective is reversed. *Viso* is derived from *visum*, the past participle of the Latin verb *vidēre* (to see), and literally means "that which is seen." The *visa* is the confirmation that a person has been examined by institutionally authorised others as to certain characteristics necessary to allow that person enter a country.

Based on this model, it is possible to further develop the concept of subjectivity in the interplay between perspectives and frames. The concept of subjectivity, as pure transcendence of the subject, allows the paradox of always being oneself and yet always being different depending on the different social contexts to be articulated in a coherent way. With the husband or wife, one is a different person than with the professor, the student, or the cashier in the supermarket. Subjectivity can be seen as the fulcrum, (i.e., as self-givenness and mystery) where the different perspectives of the play of interpretations, which constitutes intrapersonal and interpersonal life, converge and diverge.

Every human being is immersed in a network of relationships and develops within this network. Each relationship develops within a cultural, social, and emotional framework. Relationships are organized from the perspective of the subject: There are people we want to be close to and those we keep at a distance. *Close* and *far* are deictic categories of language that can be applied to intersubjective relations. Perspective also contains a moment of time: There are people we would rush at immediately, others we keep waiting. The phenomenology of these relations can multiply infinitely because perspectives and frames are potentially infinite.

The phenomenology of schizophrenia shows that not all people have subjectivity that developed in the same way. If we wanted to define human intelligence, we could say that it is the ability to shift quickly and easily from one frame to another and to change perspectives. And in this way, life causes people to deal with change and respond in an appropriate way. Knowing how to adapt and how to reinvent oneself is the most difficult and at the same time fascinating skill to acquire.

Not everyone is able to integrate the different representations of themselves, the different perspectives, and the different frames in a confident way. There are people with broader and narrower horizons. Some people are able to combine large projects of life with attention to the everyday and the ephemeral: The frames and perspectives vary in breadth.

Following everyday language, we have come to a point where heterogeneous interpretations of the human being and subjectivity meet, for instance, in expressions such as *cultural frame* (Appadurai, 2001, 2013), *cognitive frame* (Hannerz, 1996), *experiential frame* (Goffman, 1974), *action frame* (Esser, 2001), *intersubjective dialogical thinking* (Buber, 1954; Ebner, 1921; Kimura, 2013; Lévinas, 1961, 1991; Rosenzweig, 1921), and *intersubjective dialogical thinking and identity* (Devereux, 1967; Jullien, 2017; Mauss, 1938; Ricœur, 1996). From here we take up the notion of Subjectivation.

7.3 Subjectivation

Reflections on the personal pronoun *I*, on the ontological relationship between *I* and *you*, on the relationships to one's own person, and to other persons form a basis for the phenomenological analysis of the impaired subjectivity in schizophrenia.

German psychopathology uses the term *Subjektivierung*, (*Subjectivation*), to define the pathological form of *subjectivity*. English psychopathological terminology uses the terms *subjectivation* and *subjectivity*.

Subjectivation is explained by Kraepelin's frequently quoted beautiful metaphor according to which the consciousness of the schizophrenic is an "orchestra without a conductor" (Kraepelin, 1913, p. 668). This metaphor falls short. In Kraepelin's work, only a paralyzed intentional activity of the subject is shown, i.e., a *psychological impairment*. In this work, on the other hand, we illustrate an *ontological impairment*. Subjectivation only partially allows the transcending of frames and perspectives, as could be shown in the model of the three dimensions.

This model of the three dimensions of the person, which are understood through the terms *volto*, *faccia*, and *viso*, is consistent with the interpretation of subjectivity provided by Fuchs in his article on subjectivity and schizophrenia (Fuchs, 2012). After describing the pre-reflexive and reflexive forms of self-experience, Fuchs shows "four aspects of basic disturbance" in schizophrenia:

(a) A weakening of the primary bodily self-experience.
(b) A disturbance of the implicit functions of the body, resulting in an alienation of perception and action (ecological self).
(c) A disturbance of interpersonal contact with others (social self).
(d) Finally, there is a disturbance at the level of the personal self that affects the "eccentric position" (Plessner 1975) and thus the demarcation between the self and the other. (Fuchs, 2012, p. 891; source in German).

The four aspects of the schizophrenic disorder listed above summarize the clinical manifestations of schizophrenia. Points (a and b) concern the basic layers of the ego and the world in which the ego enters into relationship with itself and the outside world. Points (c and d) concern the schizophrenia patients' relationships to the social framework and their relationships to the play of perspectives between them and others. The subjectivity impaired in schizophrenia, i.e., the subjectivation of the schizophrenic ego, shows a subject not strong enough to handle perspectives flexibly and to transcend itself. Schizophrenia as conceptualized in this work is in line with the interpretation of schizophrenia proposed by Fuchs (2012): This disorder is conceptualized as a basal disorder of self-experience. The abovementioned loss of center corresponds to what is called in phenomenology *disembodiment* (cf. the overview in Fuchs, 2012, p. 891). As a direct consequence of this loss or, in other words, as a direct expression of basal and disembodied self-disturbance, schizophrenia manifests itself not only in a weakening of the primary bodily self-experience but also in the impaired forms of both the ecological self and the social self (Fuchs, 2012, p. 891). The impaired reflexivity of the human being here manifests itself through inability to switch and, at the same time, distinguish between embodied perspectives and virtual perspectives of others (Fuchs, 2012, p. 897). It follows that both the pre-reflexive and reflexive dimensions of subjectivity are affected by schizophrenia.

Because of subjectivation, the individuals with schizophrenia are unable to articulate coherently and adequately the multiple frames and perspectives in which we are involved on a daily basis.

Other central symptoms of schizophrenia have not been addressed in this work: hallucinations, delirium, some forms of eroticism, or other bizarre behaviors. It could be the task of future studies to examine these phenomena within the subjectivity-frame- perspective theory. It is to be asked whether the bizarre behaviors or hallucinations can be interpreted as manifestations of the loss of the ability to deal with frames. The inability to deal with frames means being unable to clearly see and share the distinctions of others between the real and the imaginary, between the moral and the immoral, between the legal and the illegal, between the habitual and the unusual. The boundlessness of delusion should now be able to be interpreted as a boundlessness of frame and perspective.

Because schizophrenia destroys the ability to act within shared frames and perspectives, schizophrenia is a disorder of being with.

8 Positioning of This Work in the Development of Phenomenological Psychopathology

The validity of the triad *subjectivity, frame*, *perspective* is in principle not unique to the specific field of schizophrenia. Since the correlation between these three terms corresponds to a general principle, it could be used in other areas of psychopathology as well. An elementary as well as clear example is depression. This mental disorder, which belongs to the affective disorders, reveals a weakening of the ego, i.e., of stable and powerful subjectivity on the one hand and a more or less accentuated absence of perspective and frame on the other hand. According to this interpretation, the classical symptoms of depression could be interpreted from a new perspective: decreased self-esteem; feelings of insufficiency, of guilt, and of inferiority; avolition; and increased fatigue are symptoms or impairments of subjectivity; suicidal thoughts or actions, hopelessness, and a negative and pessimistic perspective on the future are to be understood as lack of perspective and meaninglessness of life; helplessness and loss of relating are to be understood as framelessness. The frame plays an inclusive function as it frames different elements together: The social and relational frame is almost absent in depression as individuals with depression tend to self-isolate and withdraw. The powerful subjectivity of the healthy person, which sets an inclusive social frame, seems to be impaired to a high degree in depression.

P. Parisi, *A Phenomenological Interpretation of Schizophrenia*,
https://doi.org/10.1007/978-3-031-67860-8_8

9 Limitation of the Approach

The method guiding the approach of this research on the symptomatology of schizophrenia is phenomenological, although a technical-scientific study-based approach to the themes and clinical manifestations of schizophrenia should be subjected to an in-depth analysis because the state of research shows some lack of scientific description of the understanding of irony in individuals with schizophrenia.

Although the phenomenological method plays a very relevant role, since with it the study of schizophrenia is based on technically based experiments and analyses, it remains at the level of description, without offering effective explanations about the organic and neuroscientific causes of symptomatology.

Another limitation of our approach and of the analysis of artworks treated here phenomenologically is the small number of drawings and other art representations. Further statistical analysis based on a larger quantity of artworks is therefore recommended.

P. Parisi, *A Phenomenological Interpretation of Schizophrenia*,
https://doi.org/10.1007/978-3-031-67860-8_9

References

Addington, J., & Addington, D. (1998). Facial affect recognition and information in schizophrenia and bipolar disorder. *Schizophrenia Research, 32*, 171–181.

Adornetti, I. (2018). *Patologie del linguaggio e della comunicazione* (p. 125). Carocci.

Agarwal, S. M., Danivas, V., Amaresha, A. C., Shibakumar, V., Kalmady, S. V., Bose, A., Narayanaswamy, J. C., & Venkatasubramanian, G. (2015). Cognitive mapping deficits in schizophrenia: Evidence from clinical correlates of visuospatial transformation. *Psychiatry Research, 228*(3), 304–311.

Agarwal, S. M., Shivakumar, V., Kalmady, S. V., Daniva, V., Amaresha, A. C., Bose, A., Narayanaswamy, J. C., Amorim, M. A., & Venkatasubramanian, G. (2017). Neural correlates of a perspective-taking task using in a realistic three-dimensional environment based task: A pilot functional magnetic resonance imaging study. *Clinical Psychopharmacology and Neuroscience, 15*, 276–277.

Amorim, M. A. (2003). "What is my avatar seeing?": The coordination of "out-of-body" and "embodied" perspectives for scene recognition across views. *Visual Cognition, 10*, 157–199.

Andreasen, N. C. (1979). Thought, language and communication disorders: 2 diagnostic significance. *Archives of General Psychiatry, 36*, 1325–1330.

Appadurai, A. (2001). *Modernità in polvere*. Raffaello Cortina Editore.

Appadurai, A. (2013). *Il futuro come fatto culturale. Saggi sulla condizione globale*. Raffaello Cortina Ed.

Aristotele. (2000). *Poetica*. Bompiani.

Aristotele. (2014). *Retorica*. Bompiani.

Arzouan, Y., Goldstein, A., & Faust, M. (2007). Brainwaves are stethoscopes: ERP correlates of novel metaphor comprehension. *Brain Research, 1160*, 69–81.

Astington, J. W., Harris, P. L., & Olson, D. R. (1988). *Developing theories of mind*. Cambridge University Press.

Austin, J. (1962a). *Zur Theorie der Sprechakte: (How to do things with words)*. Reclam.

Austin, J. (1962b). *Come fare cose con le parole*. Marietti Editore.

Backus, B. T., Fleet, D. J., Parker, A. J., & Heeger, D. J. (2001). Human cortical activity correlates with stereoscopic depth perception. *Journal of Neurophysiology, 86*, 2054–2068.

Baillargeon, R., Scott, R. M., & He, Z. (2010). False-belief understanding in infants. *Trends in Cognitive Sciences, 14*(3), 110–118.

Bambini, V. (2017). *Il cervello pragmatico* (pp. 57–58). Carocci.

Bar, M., Kassam, K. S., Ghuman, A. S., Boshyan, J., Schmid, A. M., Dale, A. M., Hämäläinen, M. S., Marinkovic, K., Schacter, D. L., Rosen, B. R., & Halgren, E. (2006). Top-down facilitation of visual recognition. *Proceedings of the National Academy of Sciences, 103*(2), 449–454.

Barbato, M., Collinson, S. L., & Casagrande, M. (2012). Altered depth perception is associated with presence of schizotypal personality traits. *Cognitive Neuropsychiatry, 17*, 115–132.

P. Parisi, *A Phenomenological Interpretation of Schizophrenia*, https://doi.org/10.1007/978-3-031-67860-8

Baron-Cohen, S., Leslie, A. M., & Frith, U. (1985). Does the autistic child have a theory of mind? *Cognition, 21*(I), 37–46.
Barth, A., & Kufferle, B. (2001). Development of a proverb test for assessment of concrete thinking problems in schizophrenic patients. *Nervenarzt, 72*, 853–858.
Basnáková, J. (2013). Beyond the language given: The neural correlates of inferring speaker meaning. *Cerebral Cortex, 24*(10), 2572–2578.
Bateson, G. (1972). *Verso un'ecologia della mente* (pp. 218–235). Adelphi, 413-428.
Bauman, Z. (1999). *Modernità liquida*. Laterza.
Bentin, S., Allison, T., Puce, A., Perez, E., & McCarthy, G. (1996). Electrophysiological studies of face perception in humans. *Journal of Cognitive Neuroscience, 8*, 551–565.
Benveniste, É. (1965a). Langage et expérience humaine. *Diogenes, 1965*(51), 9.
Benveniste, É. (1965b). Language and human experience. *Diogenes, 13*(51), 1–12.
Benveniste, É. (1966). *Essere di parola. Semantica, soggettività, cultura* (p. 114). Mondadori.
Bergson, H. (1889). *Saggio sui dati immediati della coscienza*. Raffaello Cortina Editore.
Bergson, H. (1896). *Materia e memoria*. Laterza.
Bergson, H. (1907). *L'evoluzione creatrice*. Raffaello Cortina Editore.
Bestelmeyer, P. E. G., Tatler, B. W., Phillips, L. H., Fraser, G., Benson, P. J., & Clair, D. S. (2006). Global visual scanning abnormalities in schizophrenia and bipolar disorder. *Schizophrenia Research, 87*, 212–222.
Bianchi, C. (2009). *Pragmatica cognitiva. I meccanismi della comunicazione*. Laterza.
Birdwhistell, R. (1970). *Kinesics and context: Essays on body motion communication*. University of Pennsylvania Press.
Black, M. (1954). Metaphor. *Proceedings of the Aristotelian Society, 55*, 273–294.
Black, M. (1962). *Models and metaphors*. Cornell University Press.
Black, M. (1990). *Perplexities: Rational choice, the prisoner's dilemma, metaphor, poetic ambiguity, and other puzzles*. Cornell University Press.
Blankenburg, W. (1991). *Der Verlust der natürlichen Selbstverständlichkeit. Ein Beitrag zur Psychopathologie symptomarmer Schizophrenien* (pp. 113–115). Porodos.
Bleuler, E. (1911). *Dementia precox o il gruppo delle schizofrenie*. Carocci.
Bobrow, S., & Bell, S. (1973). On catching on to idiomatic expressions. *Memory and Cognition, I*(3), 343–346.
Boehm, G. (2007). *Wie Bilder Sinn Erzeugen. Die Macht des Zeigens* (pp. 229–242). Berlin University Press.
Borg, E. (2004). *Minimal semantics*. Clarendon Press.
Borgna, E. (1995). *Come se finesse il mondo. Il senso dell'esperienza schizofrenica* (pp. 108–109). Feltrinelli.
Bosia, M., Riccaboni, R., & Poletti, S. (2012). Neurofunctional correlates of theory of mind deficits in schizophrenia. *Current Topics in Medicinal Chemistry, 12*, 2284–2304.
Boudewyn, M. A., Carter, C. S., Long, D. L., Traxler, M. J., Lesh, T. A., Mangun, G. R., & Swaab, T. Y. (2017). Language context processing deficits in schizophrenia: The role of attentional engagement. *Neuropsychologia, 96*, 262–273.
Breitmeyer, B. G. (1984). *Visual masking: An integrative approach*. Oxford University Press.
Brüne, M. (2003). Theory of mind and the role of IQ in chronic disorganized schizophrenia. *Schizophrenia Research, 60*, 57–64.
Brune, M., & Bodenstein, L. (2005). Proverb comprehension reconsidered – "theory of mind" and the pragmatic use of language in schizophrenia. *Schizophrenia Research, 75*, 233–239.
Buber, M. (1954). *Il principio dialogico e altri saggi*. Cinisello Balsamo (Milano): San Paolo.
Burgess, N., Maguire, E. A., Spiers, H. J., & O'Keefe, J. (2001). A temporoparietal and prefrontal network for retrieving the spatial context of lifelike events. *NeuroImage, 14*, 625–641.
Butler, C. (2002). *Postmodernism: A very short introduction*. Oxford University Press.
Butler, P. D., Abeles, I. Y., Weiskopf, N. G., Tambini, A., Jalbrzikowski, M., Legatt, M. E., Zemon, V., Loughead, J., Gur, R. C., & Javitt, D. C. (2009). Sensory contributions to impaired emotion processing in schizophrenia. *Schizophrenia Bulletin, 35*, 1095–1107.

Butler, P. D., & Javitt, D. C. (2005). Early-stage visual processing deficits in schizophrenia. *Current Opinion in Psychiatry, 18*, 151–157.

Butler, P. D., Martinez, A., Foxe, J., Dongsoo, K., Vance, Z., Silipo, G., Mahoney, J., Shpaner, M., Jalbrzikowski, M., & Javit, D. C. (2007). Subcortical visual dysfunction in schizophrenia drives secondary cortical impairments. *Brain, 130*, 417–430.

Butler, P. D., Schechter, I., Zemon, V., Schwartz, S. G., Greenstein, V. C., Gordon, J., Schroeder, C. E., & Javitt, D. C. (2001). Dysfunction of early-stage visual processing in schizophrenia. *The American Journal of Psychiatry, 158*, 1126–1133.

Butler, P. D., Silverstein, S. M., & Dakin, S. C. (2008). Visual perception and its impairment in schizophrenia. *Biological Psychiatry, 64*(1), 40–47.

Butler, P. D., Zemon, V., Schechter, I., Saperstein, A. M., Hoptman, M. J., & Lim, K. O. (2005). Early-stage visual processing and cortical amplification deficits in schizophrenia. *Archives of General Psychiatry, 62*(5), 495–504.

Cacciari, C. (1991). *Teorie della metafora. L'acquisizione, la comprensione e l'uso del linguaggio figurato* (p. 3). Raffaello Cortina Editore.

Cappelen, H., & Lepore, E. (2005). *Insensitive semantics: A defense of semantic minimalism and speech act pluralism*. Blackwell.

Carston, R. (2002). *Thoughts and utterances: The pragmatics of explicit communication*. Blackwell.

Cavezian, C., Danckert, J., Lerond, J., Dalery, J., d'Amato, T., & Saoud, M. (2007). Visual-perceptual abilities in healthy controls, depressed patients, and schizophrenia patients. *Brain and Cognition, 64*, 257–264.

Caviglia, G., & Perrella, R. (2009). *La schizofrenia: Diagnosi, teorie, terapie*. Carocci.

Cazzullo, C. L., & Sini, C. (1984). *Fenomenologia: Filosofia e psichiatria*. Elsevier.

Ceccherini-Nelli, A., & Crow, T. J. (2003). Disintegration of the components of language as the path to a revision of Bleuler's and Schneider's concepts of schizophrenia. *British Journal of Psychiatry, 182*, 233–240.

Cestari, V., Saraulli, D., Spataro, P., Lega, A., Sciarretta, A., Rezende Marques, V., & Rossi-Arnaud, C. (2013). Memory for symmetry and perceptual binding in patients with schizophrenia. *Acta Psychologica, 144*, 594–603.

Chapman, L. J. (1960). Confusion of figurative and literal usages of words by schizophrenics and brain damaged patients. *The Journal of Abnormal Psychology and Social Psychology, 60*, 412–416.

Chen, E. Y. H., Lam, L. C. W., Kan, C. S., Chan, C. K. J., Kwok, C. L., Nguyen, D. G. H., & Chen, R. Y. L. (1996). Language disorganisation in schizophrenia: Validation and assessment with a new clinical rating instrument. *Hong Kong Journal of Psychiatry, 6*, 4–13.

Chen, Y., Norton, D., & McBain, R. (2008). Can persons with schizophrenia appreciate visual art? *Schizophrenia Research, 105*, 245–251.

Chiurazzi, G. (2007). *Il postmoderno*. Mondadori.

Clark, C. M., Gosselin, F., & Goghari, V. M. (2013). Aberrant patterns of visual facial information usage in schizophrenia. *Journal of Abnormal Psychology, 122*, 513–519.

Clark, H., & Lucy, P. (1975). Understanding what is meant from what is said: A study in conversationally conveyed requests. *Journal of Verbal Learning and Verbal Behavior, 14*(I), 56–72.

Coleman, M. J., Cestnick, L., Krastoshevsky, O., Krause, V., Huang, Z., Mendell, N. R., & Levy, D. L. (2009). Schizophrenia patients show deficits in shifts of attention to different levels of global-local stimuli: Evidence for magnocellular dysfunction. *Schizophrenia Bulletin, 35*, 1108–1116.

Condray, R., & Steinhauer, S. R. (2003). Mechanisms of disrupted language comprehension in schizophrenia. *Behavioral and Brain Sciences, 26*, 87–88.

Conrad, K. (1959). *Die beginnende Schizophrenie* (pp. 63–149). Psychiatrie-Verlag.

Covington, M. A., He, C., Brown, C., Naçi, L., McClain, J. T., Fjordbak, B. S., Semple, J., & Brown, J. (2005). Schizophrenia and the structure of language: The linguist's view. *Schizophrenia Research, 77*, 85–98.

Cummings, L. (2014). *Pragmatic disorders*. Springer.

Cummings, L. (2017). *Research in clinical pragmatics*. Springer.

Cutting, J., & Murphy, D. (1990). Preference for denotative as opposed to connotative meanings in schizophrenics. *Brain and Language, 39*(3), 459–468.

Dale, R. (1968). *Louis Wain: The man who drew cats*. Kimber.

Damiani, S., & Fusar-Poli, L. (2018). The cats of Louis Wain: A thousand ways to draw one's mind. *The American Journal of Psychiatry, 175*, 315.

Darwin, C. (1872). *The expression of the emotions in man and animals*. Fontana Press.

De Bonis, M. (1997). The comprehension of metaphors in schizophrenia. *Psychopathology, 30*(3), 149–154.

De Grauwe, S. (2010). Electrophysiological insights into the processing of nominal metaphors. *Neuropsychologia, 48*(7), 1965–1984.

De Libera, A. (1984). *Introduzione alla mistica renana. Da Alberto Magno a Meister Eckhart* (p. 193). Jaca Book.

De Lisi, L. E. (2001). Speech disorder in schizophrenia: Review of the literature and exploration of its relation to the uniquely human capacity for language. *Schizophrenia Bulletin, 27*, 481–496.

De Lisi, L. E., Sakuma, M., Kushner, M., Finer, D. L., Hoff, A. L., & Crow, T. J. (1997). Anomalous cerebral asymmetry and language processing in schizophrenia. *Schizophrenia Bulletin, 23*, 255–271.

De Martino, E. (1977). *La fine del mondo. Contributo all'analisi delle apocalissi culturali* (pp. 133–140). Einaudi.

Decety, J., & Lamm, C. (2007). The role of the right temporoparietal junction in social interaction: How low-level computational processes contribute to meta-cognition. *The Neuroscientist, 13*, 580–593.

Delerue, C., Laprévote, V., Verfaillie, K., & Boucart, M. (2010). Gaze control during face exploration in schizophrenia. *Neuroscience Letters, 482*, 247.

Delis, D. C., Kiefner, M. G., & Friedlund, A. J. (1988). Visuospatial dysfunction following unilateral brain damage: Dissociation in hierarchical hemispatial analysis. *Journal of Clinical and Experimental Neuropsychology, 10*, 421–431.

Devereux, G. (1967). *La rinuncia all'identità. Una difesa contro l'annientamento*. Mimesis.

Dima, D., Dietrich, D. E., Dillo, W., & Emrich, H. M. (2010). Impaired top-down processes in schizophrenia: A DCM study of ERPs. *NeuroImage, 52*, 824–832.

Dima, D., Roiser, J. P., Dietrich, D. E., Bonnenmann, C., Lanfermann, H., Emrich, H. M., & Dillo, W. (2009). Understanding why patients with schizophrenia do not perceive the hollow-mask illusion using dynamic causal modelling. *NeuroImage, 46*, 1180–1186.

Ditman, T., Goff, D., & Kuperberg, G. (2011). Slow and steady: Sustained effects of lexico-semantic associations can medicate referential impairments in schizophrenia. *Cognitive, Affective, & Behavioral Neuroscience, 11*, 245–258.

Ditman, T., & Kuperberg, G. (2010). Building coherence: A framework for exploring the breakdown of links across boundaries in schizophrenia. *Journal of Neurolinguistics, 22*, 254–269.

Docherty, N. M., Cohen, A. S., Nienow, T. M., Dizneo, T. J., & Dangelmaier, R. E. (2003). Stability of formal thought disorder and referential communication disturbances in schizophrenia. *Journal of Abnormal Psychology, 112*, 469–475.

Docherty, N. M., De Rosa, M., & Andreasen, N. C. (1996). Communication disturbances in schizophrenia and mania. *Archives of General Psychiatry, 53*, 358–364.

Domaneschi, F. (2014). *Introduzione alla pragmatica*. Carocci.

Doniger, G. M., Foxe, J. J., Schroeder, C. E., Murray, M. M., Higgins, B. A., & Javitt, D. C. (2001). Visual perceptual learning in human object recognition areas: A repetition priming study using high-density electrical mapping. *NeuroImage, 13*, 305–313.

Doody, G. A. (1998). Theory of mind and psychoses. *Psychological Medicine, 28*, 397–405.

Dreben, E. K., Fryer, J. H., & McNair, D. M. (1995). Perceptual and conceptual information processing in schizophrenia and depression. *Perceptual and Motor Skills, 80*, 447–465.

Drury, V. M., Robinson, E. J., & Birchwood, M. (1998). "Theory of mind" skills during an acute episode of psychosis and following recovery. *Psychological Medicine, 28*, 1101–1112.

Dummet, M. (1993). *Frege: Philosophy of language*. Harvard University Press.

Ebner, F. (1921). *La parola e le realtà spirituali. Frammenti pneumatologici*. San Paolo.

Eco, U. (1999). *Die grenzen der interpretation* (p. 306). Deutscher Taschenbuch.

Eco, U. (2005). La metafora nel Medioevo latino. In A. M. Lorusso (Ed.), *Metafora e conoscenza*. Bompiani.

Eco, U. (2014). *Comunicazione soft e hard. Lectio Magistralis*. Festival della comunicazione, Camogli.

Egger, V. (1881). *La parole intérieure: Essai de psychologie descriptive*. Baillière.

Ekman, P. (2016). *Nonverbal messages: Cracking the code: My Life's pursuit*. Paul Ekman Group LLC.

Ekman, P., & Scherer, K. R. (1982). *Handbook of methods in nonverbal behavior research*. Cambridge University Press.

Emrich, H. M. (1989). A three-component-system hypothesis of psychosis. impairment of binocular depth inversion as an indicator of a functional dysequilibrium. *British Journal of Psychiatry, 155*, 37–39.

Emrich, H. M., Weber, M. M., Wendel, A., Zihl, J., von Meyer, L., & Hanisch, W. (1991). Reduced binocular depth inversion as an indicator of cannabis-induced censorship impairment. *Pharmacology Biochemistry and Behavior, 40*, 689–690.

Ervas, F., & Gola, E. (2016). *Che cos'è una metafora*. Carocci.

Esser, H. (2001). *Soziologie. Spezielle Grundlagen. Band 6: Sinn und Kultur*. Campus Verlag.

Etchamendy, N., & Bohbot, V. D. (2007). Spontaneous navigational strategies and performance in the virtual town. *Hippocampus, 17*, 595–599.

Evans, M. A., Shedden, J. M., Hevenor, S. J., & Hahn, M. C. (2000). The effect of variability of unattended information on global and local processing: Evidence for lateralization at early stages of processing. *Neuropsychologia, 38*, 225–239.

Feinberg, T. E., Rifkin, A., Schaffer, C., & Walker, E. (1986). Facial discrimination and emotional recognition in schizophrenia and affective disorders. *Archives of General Psychiatry, 43*, 276–279.

Fernandez, D., & Wilkins, A. J. (2008). Uncomfortable images in art and nature. *Perception, 37*(7), 1098–1113.

Fink, G. R., Halligan, P. W., Marshall, J. C., Firth, C. D., Frackowiak, R. S., & Dolan, R. J. (1996). Where in the brain does visual attention select the forest and the trees? *Nature, 382*, 626–628.

Fischer, F. (1929). Zeitstruktur und Schizophrenie. *Zeitschrift für die gesamte Neurologie und Psychiatrie, CXXI*, 544–574.

Fischer, F. (1930a). Weitere Mitteilung über das schizophrene Zeiterleben. *Neurologie et Psychiatrie, 57*, 563–564.

Fischer, F. (1930b). Raum-Zeit-Struktur und Denkstörung in der Schizophrenie. *Zeitschrift für die gesamte Neurologie und Psychiatrie, CXXIV*, 61–72.

Fraser, W. I., King, K. M., Thomas, P., & Kendell, R. E. (1986). The diagnosis of schizophrenia by language analysis. *British Journal of Psychiatry, 148*, 275–278.

Frith, C. D. (1992). *The cognitive neuropsychology of schizophrenia* (p. 80). Psychology Press.

Frith, C. D., & Corcoran, R. (1996). Exploring "theory of mind" in people with schizophrenia. *Psychological Medicine, 26*, 521–530.

Frith, C. D., & Johnstone, E. (2003). *Schizophrenia. A very short introduction* (p. 30). Oxford University Press.

Frith, U. (1989). *Autism: Explaining the enigma* (p. 83). Blackwell Publishers.

Fuchs, T. (2007). The temporal structure of intentionality and its disturbance in schizophrenia. *Psychopathology, 40*, 231.

Fuchs, T. (2012). Selbst und Schizophrenie. *Deutsche Zeitschrift für Philosophie, 60*, 887.

Fuchs, T. (2013). Temporality and psychopathology. *Phenomenology and the Cognitive Sciences, 12*, 75–104.

Fuchs, T. (2017a). The 'as if' function and its loss in schizophrenia. In M. Summa, T. Fuchs, & L. Vanzago (Eds.), *Imagination and social perspectives. Approaches from phenomenology and psychopathology* (p. 87). Routledge.

Fuchs, T. (2017b). Time and events: On the phenomenology of temporal experience in schizophrenia (ancillary article to EAWE domain 2). *Psychopathology, 50*, 68–74.

Gaebel, W., Ulrich, G., & Frick, K. (1987). Visuomotor performance of schizophrenic patients and normal controls in a picture viewing task. *Biological Psychiatry, 22*, 1227–1237.

Galimberti, U. (1979). *Psichiatria e fenomenologia*. Feltrinelli.

Gavilán Ibáñey, J. M., & García-Albea Ristol, J. E. (2011). Theory of mind and language comprehension in schizophrenia: Poor mindreading affects figurative language comprehension beyond intelligence deficits. *Journal of Neurolinguistics, 24*, 54–69.

Genette, G. (1972). La Rhétorique restreinte. In G. Genette (Ed.), *Figures III* (pp. 21–40). Seuil.

Gensini, S. (2004). Metaphor according to Gianbattista Vico: An exemplary case of iconic theory. *Logos and Language, 5*, 35–38.

Gibbs, R. W. (1994). *The poetics of mind: Figurative thought, language, and understanding*. Cambridge University Press.

Gibbs, R. W. (2001). Evaluating contemporary models of figurative language understanding. *Metaphor and Symbol, 16*(3), 317–333.

Gibbs, R. W. (2008). *The Cambridge handbook of metaphor and thought*. Cambridge University Press.

Giddens, A. (1990). *Le conseguenze della modernità. Fiducia e rischio, sicurezza e pericolo*. Il Mulino.

Gildea, P., & Glucksberg, S. (1983). On understanding metaphor: The role of context. *Journal of Verbal Learning and Verbal Behavior, 22*(5), 577–590.

Glucksberg, S. (2001). *Understanding figurative language: From metaphors to idioms*. Oxford University Press.

Goffman, E. (1959). *The presentation of self in everyday life*. Doubleday.

Goffman, E. (1974). *Frame analisys. L'organizzazione dell'esperienza*. Armando Editore.

Gold, R., Butler, P., Revheim, N., Leitman, D. I., Hansen, J. A., Gur, R. C., Kantrowitz, J. T., Laukka, P., Juslin, P. N., Silipo, G. S., & Javitt, D. C. (2012). Auditory emotion recognition impairments in schizophrenia: Relationship to acoustic features and cognition. *The American Journal of Psychiatry, 169*, 424–432.

Gordon, E., Coyle, S., Anderson, J., Healy, P., Cordaro, J., Latimer, C., & Meares, R. (1992). Eye movement response to a facial stimulus in schizophrenia. *Biological Psychiatry, 31*, 626–629.

Graham, D., & Meng, M. (2011). Altered spatial frequency content in paintings by artists with schizophrenia. *Perception, 2*, 1–9.

Graham, D. J., & Field, D. J. (2007). Statistical regularities of art images and natural scenes: Spectra, sparseness and nonlinearities. *Spatial Vision, 21*, 149–164.

Graham, D. J., & Field, D. J. (2008). Variation in intensity statistics for representational and abstract art, and for art from the Eastern and Western hemispheres. *Perception, 37*, 1341–1352.

Graham, D. J., & Redies, C. (2010). Statistical regularities in art: Relations with visual coding and perception. *Vision Research, 50*, 1503–1509.

Green, M. F. & Bearden, C. E. & & Cannon, T. D. & Fiske, A. P. & Hellemann, G. S. & Horan, W. et al. (2012). Social cognition in schizophrenia. Schizophrenia Bulletin, 38, 854–864.

Green, M. J., Nuechterlein, K. H., & Mintz, J. (1994). Backward masking in schizophrenia and mania, II: Specifying the visual channels. *Archives of General Psychiatry, 51*, 945–951.

Green, M. J., Williams, L. M., & Davidson, D. (2003). Visual scanpaths to threat-related faces in deluded schizophrenia. *Psychiatry Research, 119*, 271–285.

Green, M. J., Williams, L. M., & Hemsley, D. R. (2000). Cognitive theories of delusion formation: The contribution of visual scanpath research. *Cognitive Neuropsychiatry, 5*, 63–74.

Gregory, R. L. (1970). *The intelligent eye*. Weidenfeld & Nicolson.

Grice, P. (1957). Meaning. *The Philosophical Review, 66*, 377–388.

Gruzelier, J. H., Wilson, L., Liddiard, D., Peters, E., & Pusavsat, L. (1999). Cognitive asymmetry patterns in schizophrenia: Active and withdrawn syndromes and sex differences as moderators. *Schizophrenia Bulletin, 25*, 349–362.

Hahn, B., Robinson, B. M., Harvey, A. N., & Kaiser, S. T. (2012). Visuospatial attention in schizophrenia: Deficits in broad monitoring. *Journal of Abnormal Psychology, 1*, 119–128.

Halliday, M., & Hasan, R. (1976). *Cohesion in English*. Longman.
Handke, P. (1970). *Die Angst des Tormanns beim Elfmeter* (p. 119). Suhrkamp.
Handke, P. (2020). *The goalkeeper's anxiety at the penalty kick*. Penguin Books Ltd.
Hannerz, U. (1996). *La diversità culturale*. Il Mulino.
Hegel, G. W. F. (1820). *Grundlinien der Philosophie des Rechts*. Suhrkamp.
Heidegger, M. (1927). *Sein und Zeit*. Max Niemeyer Verlag.
Heimberg, C., Gur, R. E., Erwin, R. J., Shtasel, D. L., & Gur, R. C. (1992). Facial emotion discrimination: III. Behavioural findings in schizophrenia. *Psychiatry Research, 42*, 253–265.
Heinze, H. J., Hinrichs, H., Scholz, M., Burchert, W., & Mangun, G. R. (1998). Neural mechanisms of global and local processing. A combined PET and ERP study. *Journal of Cognitive Neuroscience, 10*, 485–498.
Hella, P., Niemi, J., Hintikka, J., Otsa, L., Tirkonnen, J.-M., & Koponen, H. (2013). Disordered semantic activation in disorganized discourse in schizophrenia: A new pragma-linguistic tool for structure and meaning reconstruction. *International Journal of Language & Communication Disorders, 48*(3), 320–328.
Henemann, G. M., Brachmann, A., & Redies, C. (2017). Statistical image properties in works from the prinzhorn collection of artists with schizophrenia. *Frontiers in Psychiatry, 8*, 273.
Holm-Hadulla, R. (1982). Der Konkretismus als Ausdruck schizophrenen Denkens, Sprechens und Verhaltens. *Der Nervenarzt, 53*, 524–529.
Holm-Hadulla, R. (1988). Über den strukturellen Zusammenhang schizophrener Denk- und Sprachstörungen mit wahnhaften Erleben und Abwandlungen der Intentionalität. *Fortschritte der Neurologie-Psychiatrie, 56*, 1–7.
Holm-Hadulla, R., & Haug, F. (1984). Die interpretation von Sprichwörtern als klinische Methode zur Erfassung schizophrener Denk-, Sprach-, und Symbolisationsstörungen. *Der Nervenarzt, 55*, 496–503.
Hooker, C., & Park, S. (2002). Emotion processing and its relationship to social functioning in schizophrenia patients. *Psychiatry Research, 112*, 41–50.
Husserl, E. (1928). *Zur Phänomenologie des inneren Zeitbewusstseins* (p. 22). Felix Meiner.
Husserl, E. (1966). Analysen zur passiven synthesis. In *Aus Vorlesungs und Forschungsmanuskripten 1918-1926*. Martinus Nijhoff.
Husserl, E. (2019). *The phenomenology of internal time-consciousness*. Indiana University Press.
Iacoboni, M., & Dapretto, M. (2006). The mirror neuron system and the consequences of its dysfunction. *Nature Reviews Neuroscience, 7*, 942–951.
Iakimova, G. (2005). ERPs of metaphoric, literal, and incongruos semantic processing in schizophrenia. *Psychophysiology, 42*, 380–390.
Ikeda, C., Kirino, E., Inoue, R., & Arai, H. (2011). Event-related potential study of illusory contour perception in schizophrenia. *Neuropsychobiology, 64*(4), 231–238.
Imbo, I., Szmalec, A., & Vandierendonck, A. (2009). The role of structure on age-related increases in visuo-spatial span performance. *Psychology Belgium, 49*, 275–291.
Inhoff, A. W., Lima, S. D., & Carroll, P. J. (1984). Contextual effects on metaphor comprehension in reading. *Memory & Cognition, 12*(6), 558–567.
Itier, R. J., & Batty, M. (2009). Neural bases of eye and gaze processing: The core of social cognition. *Neuroscience & Biobehavioral Reviews, 33*, 843–863.
James, W. (1890). *The principles of psychology*. Harvard University Press.
Jameson, F. (1989). *Postmodernism: Or, the cultural logic of late capitalism*. Duke University Press.
Janus, R. A., & Bever, T. G. (1985). Processing of metaphoric language: An investigation of the three-stage model of metaphor comprehension. *Journal of Psycholinguistic Research, 14*(5), 473–487.
Johnson, S. C., Lowery, N., Kohler, C., & Turetsky, B. I. (2005). Global-local visual processing in schizophrenia: Evidence for an early visual processing deficit. *Biological Psychiatry, 58*, 937–946.
Joyce, J. (1939). *Finnegans Wake*. Mondadori.
Jullien, F. (2017). *Il gioco dell'esistenza. De-coincidenza e libertà*. Feltrinelli.

Kantrowitz, J. T., Butler, P. D., Schechter, I., Silipo, G., & Javitt, D. C. (2009). Seeing the world dimly: The impact of early visual deficits on visual experience in schizophrenia. *Schizophrenia Bulletin, 35*, 1089.
Kasanin, J. S. (1944). *Language and thought in schizophrenia*. University of California Press.
Keane, B. P., Silverstein, S. M., Wang, Y., & Papathomas, T. V. (2013). Reduced depth inversion illusions in schizophrenia are state-specific and occur for multiple object types and viewing conditions. *Journal of Abnormal Psychology, 122*(2), 506–512.
Keane, B. P., Silverstein, S. M., Wang, Y., Roché, M. W., & Papathomas, T. V. (2016). Seeing more clearly through psychosis: Depth inversion illusion are normal in bipolar disorder but reduced in schizophrenia. *Schizophrenia Research, 176*(2), 485–492.
Kemps, E. (2001). Complexity effects in visuo-spatial working memory: Implications for the role of long-term memory. *Memory, 9*, 13–27.
Keri, S. (2008). The magnocellular pathway and schizophrenia. *Visual Research, 48*, 1181–1182.
Keri, S., Kelemen, O., Benedek, G., & Janka, Z. (2004). Vernier threshold in patients with schizophrenia and their unaffected siblings. *Neuropsychology, 18*, 537–542.
Kim, C. Y. (2013). *James Turrell: A retrospective*. Prestel.
Kimchi, R. (1992). Primacy of wholistic processing and global/local paradigm: A critical review. *Psychological Bulletin, 112*, 24–38.
Kimura, B. (1992). *Scritti di psicopatologia fenomenologica*. Giovanni Fioriti Editore.
Kimura, B. (2013). *Tra. Per una fenomenologia dell'incontro*. Il pozzo di Giacobbe.
King, K., Fraser, W. I., Thomas, P., & Kendell, R. E. (1990). Re-examination of the language of psychotic subjects. *British Journal of Psychiatry, 156*, 211–215.
Kircher, T. T. J., Oh, T. M., Brammer, M. J., & McGuire, P. K. (2005). Neural correlates of syntax production in schizophrenia. *British Journal of Psychiatry, 186*, 209–214.
Koethe, D., Kranaster, L., Hoyer, C., Gross, S., Neatby, M. A., Schulze-Lutter, F., Ruhrmann, S., Klosterkötter, J., Hellmich, M., & Leweke, F. M. (2009). Binocular depth inversion as a paradigm of reduced visual information processing in prodromal state, antipsychotic-naïve and treated schizophrenia. *European Archives of Psychiatry and Clinical Neuroscience, 259*, 195–202.
Kohler, C. G., Bilker, W., Hagendoorn, M., Gur, R. E., & Gur, R. C. (2000). Emotion recognition deficit in schizophrenia: Association with symptomatology and cognition. *Biological Psychiatry, 48*, 127–136.
Kojima, T., Matsushima, E., Ando, K., Ando, H., Sakurada, M., Ohta, K., Moriya, H., & Schimazono, Y. (1992). Exploratory eye-movements and neuropsychological tests in schizophrenic-patients. *Schizophrenia Bulletin, 18*, 85–94.
Kövecses, Z. (2000). *Metaphor and emotion*. Cambridge University Press.
Kövecses, Z. (2002). *Metaphor: A practical introduction*. Oxford University Press.
Kövecses, Z. (2005). *Metaphor in culture: Universality and variation*. Cambridge University Press.
Kraepelin, E. (1913). *Klinische psychiatrie, Teil 2* (8th ed., p. 668). Barth.
Kuperberg, G. R., Kreher, D. A., & Ditman, T. (2010). What can event-related potentials tell us about language, and perhaps even thought, in schizophrenia? *International Journal of Psychophysiology, 75*, 66–76.
Kurylo, D. D., Pasternak, R., Silipo, G., Javitt, D. C., & Butler, P. D. (2007). Perceptual organization by proximity and similarity in schizophrenia. *Schizophrenia Research, 95*, 205–214.
Kurz, G. (1997). *Metapher, allegorie, symbol*. Vandenhoeck und Ruprecht.
Kutas, M., & Hillyard, S. A. (1980). Reading senseless sentences: Brain potentials reflect semantic incongruity. *Science, 207*, 203–205.
Lai, V. T., Curran, T., & Menn, L. (2009). Comprehending conventional and novel metaphors: An ERP study. *Brain Research, 1284*, 145–155.
Lakoff, G., & Johnson, M. (1980). *Metaphors we live by*. University of Chicago.
Lamb, M. R., & Robertson, L. C. (1988). The processing of hierarchical stimuli: Effects of retinal locus, locational uncertainty, and stimulus identity. *Perception & Psychophysics, 44*, 172–181.

Lambrey, S., Amorim, M. A., Samson, S., Noulhiane, M., Hasboun, D., Dupont, S., Baulac, M., & Berthoz, A. (2008). Distinct visual perspective-taking strategies involve the left and right medial temporal lobe structure differently. *Brain, 131*, 523–534.

Landert, M. (2011). *Weltensammler. Internationale Aussenseiterkunst der Gegenwart* (p. 293). Benteli.

Landgraf, S., Amado, I., Purkhart, R., Ries, J., Olié, J.-P., & van der Meer, E. (2011). Visuo-spatial cognition in schizophrenia: Confirmation of a preference for local information processing. *Schizophrenia Research, 127*, 165.

Langdon, R. (1997). Defective self and/or other mentalising in schizophrenia: A cognitive neuropsychological approach. *Cognitive Neuropsychiatry, 2*, 167–193.

Langdon, R. (2001). Mentalising, executive planning, and disengagement in schizophrenia. *Cognitive Neuropsychiatry, 6*, 81–108.

Langdon, R. (2002). Disturbed communication in schizophrenia: The role of poor pragmatics and poor theory-of-mind. *Psychological Medicine, 32*, 1273–1284.

Langdon, R., Coltheart, M., Ward, P. B., & Catts, S. V. (2001). Visual and cognitive perspective-taking impairments in schizophrenia: A failure of allocentric simulation? *Cognitive Neuropsychiatry, 6*, 241–269.

Langdon, R., Davies, M., & Coltheart, M. (2002). Understanding minds and understanding communicated meanings in schizophrenia. *Mind & Language, 17*, 1273–1284.

Lausberg, H. (1949). *Elemente der literarischen Rhetorik* (p. 237). Max Hueber.

Lévinas, E. (1961). *Totalità e infinito. Saggio sull'esteriorità*. Jaca Book.

Lévinas, E. (1991). *Tra noi. Saggio sul pensare-all'altro*. Jaca Book.

Leweke, F. M., Schneider, U., Radwan, M., Schmidt, E., & Emrich, H. M. (2000). Different effects of nabilone and cannabidiol on binocular depth inversion in man. *Pharmacology Biochemistry and Behavior, 66*, 175–181.

Leweke, F. M., Schneider, U., Thies, M., Münte, T. F., & Emrich, H. M. (1999). Effects of synthetic Δ^9-tetrahydrocannabinol on binocular depth inversion of natural and artificial objects in man. *Psychopharmacology, 142*, 230–235.

Liszkowski, U., Carpenter, M., & Tomasello, M. (2008). Twelve-month-olds communicate helpfully and appropriately for knowledgeable and ignorant partners. *Cognition, 108*(3), 732–739.

Lo Piparo, F. (2003). *Aristotele e il linguaggio. Cosa fa di una lingua una lingua*. Laterza.

Lorusso, A. M. (2005). *Metafora e conoscenza*. Bompiani.

Loughland, C. M., Williams, L. M., & Gordon, E. (2002). Visual scanpaths to positive and negative facial emotions in an outpatient schizophrenia sample. *Schizophrenia Research, 55*, 159–170.

Loughland, C. M., Williams, L. M., & Harris, A. W. (2004). Visual scanpath dysfunction in first-degree relatives of schizophrenia probands: Evidence for a vulnerability marker? *Schizophrenia Research, 67*, 11–21.

Lowen, A. (1958). *Il linguaggio del corpo*. Feltrinelli.

Luft, S., & Wehrle, M. (2017). *Husserl-Handbuch: Leben-Werk-Wirkung*. Metzler.

Lyotard, J.-F. (1979). *La condizione postmoderna. Rapporto sul sapere*. Feltrinelli.

Manetti, G. (2005). *Aristotele e la metafora. Conoscenza, similarità, azione, enunciazione*. Laterza.

Mangoni, L. (2013). *Civiltà della crisi. Cultura e politica in Italia tra Otto e Novecento*. Viella Libreria Editrice.

Manor, B. R., & Gordon, E. (2003). Defining the temporal threshold for ocular fixation in free-viewing visocognitive tasks. *Journal of Neuroscience Methods, 128*, 85–93.

Marchetti, A., Massaro, D., & Valle, A. (2007). Non dicevo sul serio. In *Riflessioni su ironia e psicologia*. Franco Angeli.

Martinez, A., Moses, P., Frank, L., Buxton, R., Wong, E., & Stiles, J. (1997). Hemispheric asymmetries in global and local processing: Evidence from fRMI. *NeuroReport, 8*, 1437–1457.

Marx, K. (1867). *Il capitale*. UTET.

Mauss, M. (1938). *La nozione di persona. Una categoria dello spirito*. Morcelliana.

Mazza, M. (2001). Selective impairments of theory of mind in people with schizophrenia. *Schizophrenia Research, 47*, 299–308.

McGennis, A. (1999). Louis Wain: His life, his art and his mental illness. *Irish Journal of Psychological Medicine, 16*, 27.
Merigan, W. H., & Maunsell, J. H. R. (1993). How parallel are the primate visual pathways. *Annual Review of Neuroscience, 16*, 369–402.
Merleau-Ponty, M. (1945). *Phänomenologie der Wahrnehmung* (p. 170). Walter de Gruyter & Co.
Merleau-Ponty, M. (2002). *Phenomenology of perception*. Routledge.
Minassian, A., Granholm, E., Verney, S., & Perry, W. (2005). Visual scanning deficits in schizophrenia and their relationship to executive functioning impairment. *Schizophrenia Research, 74*, 69–79.
Minkowski, E. (1927). *La schizofrenia. Psicopatologia degli schizoidi e degli schizofrenici*. Einaudi.
Minkowski, E. (1933). *Die gelebte Zeit* (p. 86). Otto Müller.
Minkowski, E. (1970). *Lived time phenomenological and psychopathological studies*. Northwestern University Press.
Minkowski, E. (1971). *Il tempo vissuto. Fenomenologia e psicopatologia*. Einaudi.
Minkowski, E., von Gebsattel, V., & Straus, E. (2013). *Antropologia e psicopatologia*. Editoriale Anicia.
Mitchley, N. J., Barber, J., Gray, J. M., Brooks, N., & Livingston, M. G. (1998). Comprehension of irony in schizophrenia. *Cognitive Neuropsychiatry, 3*, 127–138.
Mo, S. (2008). Comprehension of metaphor and irony in schizophrenia during remission: The role of theory of mind and IQ. *Psychiatry Research, 157*, 21–29.
Mohammadi, A., Hesami, E., Kargar, M., & Shams, J. (2017). Detecting allocentric and egocentric navigation deficits in patients with schizophrenia and bipolar disorder using virtual reality. *Neuropsychological Rehabilitation, 28*(3), 398–415.
Molaro, A., & Civita, A. (2012). *Binswanger e Freud. Tra psicoanalisi, psichiatria e fenomenologia*. Raffaello Cortina Editore.
Morice, R., & Ingram, J. C. L. (1982). Language analysis in schizophrenia: Diagnosis implications. *Australian and New Zealand Journal of Psychiatry, 16*, 11–21.
Morice, R., & McNicol, D. (1985). The comprehension and production of complex syntax in schizophrenia. *Cortex, 21*, 567–580.
Morice, R., & McNicol, D. (1986). Language changes in Schizophrenia: A limited replication. *Schizophrenia Bulletin, 12*, 239–251.
Mortara Garavelli, B. (1989). *Manuale di retorica* (p. 163). Bompiani.
Mossaheb, N. (2014). Comprehension of metaphors in patients with schizophrenia-spectrum disorders. *Comprehensive Psychiatry, 55*, 931.
Murray, M. M., Wylie, G. R., Higgins, B. A., Javitt, D. C., Schroeder, C. E., & Foxe, J. J. (2002). The spatiotemporal dynamics of illusory contour processing: Combined high-density electrical mapping, source analysis, and functional magnetic resonance imaging. *The Journal of Neuroscience, 22*, 5055–5073.
Muscelli, C., & Stanghellini, G. (2012). *Istantaneità. Cultura e psicopatologia della temporalità contemporanea*. FrancoAngeli.
Navon, D. (1977). Forest before trees: The precedence of global features in visual processing. *Cognitive Psychology, 9*, 353–383.
Navratil, L. (1965). *Schizophrenie und Kunst* (pp. 44–49). Fischer.
Nguyen, H. T., Isaacowitz, D. M., & Rubin, P. A. (2009). Age- and fatigue-related markers of human faces: An eye-tracking study. *Ophthalmology, 116*, 355–360.
Nietzsche, F. (1882). *Die Fröhliche Wissenschaft* (pp. 480–482). Deutsche Taschenbuch.
Nieuwland, M. S., & Van Berkum, J. J. A. (2006). When peanuts fall in love: N400 evidence for the power of discourse. *Journal of Cognitive Neuroscience, 18*(7), 1098–1111.
Nigro Covre, J. (2017). *Cubismo*. Giunti.
Nishida, Y., Hayashi, O., Iwami, T., Kimura, M., Kani, K., Ito, R., Shiino, A., & Suzuki, M. (2001). Stereopsis-processing regions in the human parieto-occipital cortex. *NeuroReport, 12*, 2259–2263.

O'Hare, L., & Hibbard, P. B. (2011). Spatial frequency and visual discomfort. *Vision Research, 51*, 1767–1777.
Ogmen, H. (1993). A neural theory of retino-cortical dynamics. *Neural Networks, 6*, 245–273.
Onishi, K. H., & Baillargeon, R. (2005). Do 15-month-old infants understand false beliefs? *Science, 308*(5719), 255–258.
Onitsuka, T., Niznikiewicz, M., Spencer, K. M., Frumin, M., Kuroki, N., Lucia, L. C., Shenton, M. E., & McCarley, R. W. (2006). Functional and structural deficits in brain regions subserving face perception in schizophrenia. *The American Journal of Psychiatry, 163*, 455–462.
Ortony, A. (1975). Why metaphors are necessary and not just nice. *Educational Theory, 25*(I), 45–53.
Ortony, A. (1979). *Metaphor and thought*. Cambridge University Press.
Parnas, J., Vianin, P., Saebye, D., Jansson, L., Volmer-Larsen, A., & Bovet, P. (2001). Visual binding abilities in the initial and advanced stages of schizophrenia. *Acta Psychiatrica Scandinavica, 103*, 171–180.
Penn, D. L., & Combs, D. (2000). Modification of affect perception deficits in schizophrenia. *Schizophrenia Research, 46*, 217–229.
Penn, D. L., Ritchie, M., Francis, J., Combs, D., & Martin, J. (2002). Social perception in schizophrenia: The role of context. *Psychiatry Research, 109*, 149–159.
Perlini, C., Marini, A., Garzitto, M., Isola, M., Cerruti, S., Marinelli, V., Rambaldelli, G., Ferro, A., Tomelleri, L., Dusi, N., Bellani, M., Tansella, M., Fabbro, F., & Brambilla, P. (2012). Linguistic production and syntactic comprehension in schizophrenia and bipolar disorder. *Acta Psychiatrica Scandinavica, 126*, 363–376.
Pfeifer, R. A. (1923). *Der Geisteskranke und sein Werk. Eine Studie über schizophrene Kunst* (p. 77). Alfred Kröner.
Phillips, M. L., & David, A. S. (1997). Visual scan paths are abnormal in deluded schizophrenics. *Neuropsychologia, 35*, 99–105.
Phillips, M. L., & David, A. S. (1998). Abnormal visual scan paths: A psychophysiological marker of delusions in schizophrenia. *Schizophrenia Research, 29*, 235–245.
Pieroni, L., Rossi-Arnaud, C., & Baddeley, A. D. (2011). What can symmetry tell us about working memory? In A. Vandierendonck & A. Szmalec (Eds.), *Spatial working memory* (pp. 145–159). Psychology Press.
Plessner H. (1975). *Die Stufen des Organischen und der Mensch: Einleitung in die philosophische Anthropologie*. Berlin, New York: De Gruyter. https://doi.org/10.1515/9783110845341
Pourtois, G., Dan, E. S., Grandjean, D., Sander, D., & Vuilleumier, P. (2005). Enhanced extrastriate visual response to bandpass spatial frequency filtered fearful faces: Time course and topographic evoked-potentials mapping. *Human Brain Mapping, 26*, 65–79.
Pragglejaz Group. (2007). MIP: A method for identifying metaphorically used words in discourse. *Metaphor and Symbol, 22*, 1–39.
Premack, D., & Woodruff, G. (1978). Does the Chimpanzee have a theory of mind? *Behavioral and Brain Sciences, I*(4), 515–526.
Proust, M. (1913). *Alla ricerca del tempo perduto*. BUR.
Proverbio, A. M., Minniti, A., & Zani, A. (1998). Electrophysiological evidence of a perceptual precedence of global vs. local visual information. *Cognitive Brain Research, 6*, 321–334.
Pynte, J. (1996). The time-course of metaphor comprehension: An event-related potential study. *Brain and Language, 55*(3), 293–316.
Raggiunti, R. (2007). *Introduzione a Husserl*. Laterza.
Ramsden Eames, E. (2013). *Bertrand Russell's theory of knowledge*. Routledge.
Rapp, M. A., Felsenheimer, A. K., Langohr, K., & Klupp, M. (2018). The comprehension of familiar and novel metaphoric meanings in schizophrenia: A pilot study. *Frontiers in Psychology, 8*, 1–11.
Rapp, M. A., Langohr, K., Mutschler, D. E., & Wild, B. (2014). Irony and proverb comprehension in schizophrenia: Do female patients dislike ironic remarks? *Schizophrenia Research and Treatment, 2014*, 841086.

Recanati, F. (2004). *Literal meaning*. Oxford University Press.
Redies, C., Amirshahi, S. A., Koch, M., & Denzler, J. (2012). PHOG-derived aesthetic measures applied to color photographs of artworks, natural scenes and objects. *Lecture Notes in Computer Science, 2012*, 7583.
Redies, C., Brachmann, A., & Wagemans, J. (2017). High entropy of edge orientations characterizes visual artworks from diverse cultural backgrounds. *Vision Research, 133*, 130–144.
Redies, C., Hasenstein, J., & Denzler, J. (2007). Fractal-like image statistics in visual art: Similarity to natural scenes. *Spatial Vision, 21*, 137–148.
Reed, A. (2019). *Slow art: The experience of looking, sacred images to James Turrell*. University of California Press.
Rennert, H. (1962). *Die Merkmale schizophrener Bildnerei*. Gustav-Fischer.
Richards, I. A. (1936). *The philosophy of rhetoric*. Oxford University Press.
Ricœur, P. (1996). *Sé come un altro*. Jaca Book.
Ristic, J., Mottron, L., Friesen, C. K., Iarocci, G., Burack, J. A., & Kingstone, A. (2005). Eyes are special but not for everyone: The case of autism. *Cognitive Brain Research, 24*, 715–718.
Rochester, S., & Martin, J. R. (1979). *Crazy talk. A study of the discourse of schizophrenic speakers* (p. 74). Plenum Press.
Rohleder, C., Koethe, D., Fritze, S., Topor, C. E., Leweke, F. M., & Hirjak, D. (2018). *Neural correlates of binocular depth inversion illusion in antipsychotic-naïve first-episode schizophrenia patients*. Springer.
Roni, R. (2016). *Victor Egger e Henri Bergson. Alle origini del flusso di coscienza*. ETS.
Rosenzweig, F. (1921). *La stella della redenzione*. Vita&Pensiero.
Röske, T. (1995). *Der Arzt als Künstler: Ästhetik und Psychotherapie bei Hans Prinzhorn (1886-1933)*. Aisthesis.
Rossetti, I., Brambilla, P., & Papagno, C. (2018). Metaphor comprehension in schizophrenic patients. *Frontiers in Psychology, 9*, 1–15.
Rossi-Arnaud, C., Pieroni, L., & Baddeley, A. D. (2006). Symmetry and binding in visuo-spatial working memory. *Neuroscience, 139*, 393–400.
Ruderman, D., & Bialek, W. (1994). Statistics of natural images – scaling in the woods. *Physical Review Letters, 73*, 814–817.
Russo Cardona, T. (2017). *Le peripezie dell'ironia. Sull'arte del rovesciamento discorsivo*. Meltemi.
Ryle, G. (1949). *Der Begriff des Geistes*. Reclam.
Ryu, H., Morita, K., Shoji, Y., Waseda, Y., & Maeda, H. (2001). Abnormal exploratory eye movements in schizophrenic patients vs healthy subjects. *Acta Neurologica Scandinavica, 104*, 369–376.
Sass, L. (1992). *Madness and modernism*. Oxford University Press.
Schapiro, M. (2003). *Tra Einstein e Picasso. Spazio-tempo, cubismo, futurismo*. Marinotti.
Schechter, I., Butler, P. D., Jalbrzikowski, M., Pasternak, R., Saperstein, A. M., & Javitt, D. C. (2006). A new dimension of sensory dysfunction: Stereopsis deficits in schizophrenia. *Biological Psychiatry, 60*, 1282–1284.
Schilder, P. (1942). *Mind: Perception and thought in their constructive aspects* (p. 217). Columbia University Press.
Schmidt, D., Krause, B. J., Weiss, P. H., Fink, G. R., Shah, N. J., Amorim, M. A., Müller, H.-W., & Berthoz, A. (2007). Visuospatial working memory and changes of the point of view in 3D space. *NeuroImage, 36*, 955–968.
Schneider, F., Gur, R. C., Gur, R. E., & Shtasel, D. L. (1995). Emotional processing in schizophrenia: Neurobehavioral probes in relation to psychopathology. *Schizophrenia Research, 17*, 67–75.
Schneider, U., Borsutzky, M., Seifert, J., Leweke, F. M., Huber, T. J., Rollnick, J. D., & Emrich, H. M. (2002). Reduced binocular depth inversion in schizophrenic patients. *Schizophrenia Research, 53*, 101–108.

Schneider, U., Leweke, F. M., Sternemann, U., Weber, M. M., & Hemrich, H. M. (1996). Visual 3D illusion: A system-theoretical approach to psychosis. *European Archives of Psychiatry and Clinical Neuroscience, 246*, 256–260.
Schürmann, E. (1998). *Ästhetische Wahrnehmung als ursprüngliche Erkenntnis: Eine kunstphilosophische Studie zum Werk von James Turrell*. Frankfurter Verlagsgruppe GmbH.
Semple, D. M., Ramsden, F., & McIntosh, A. M. (2003). Reduced binocular depth inversion in regular cannabis users. *Pharmacology Biochemistry and Behavior, 75*, 789–793.
Sergi, M. J., Rassovsky, Y., Nuechterlein, K. H., & Green, M. F. (2006). Social perception as mediator of the influence of early visual processing on functional status in schizophrenia. *The American Journal of Psychiatry, 163*, 448–454.
Severino, E. (2004). *La filosofia dai Greci al nostro tempo*. BUR.
Silver, H., & Bilker, W. B. (2015). Colour influences perception of facial emotions but this effect is impaired in healthy ageing and schizophrenia. *Cognitive Neuropsychiatry, 20*, 438–455.
Silver, H., Goodman, C., Knoll, G., & Isakov, V. (2004). Brief emotion training recognition of facial emotions in chronic schizophrenia. A pilot study. *Psychiatry Research, 128*, 147–154.
Silver, H., Goodman, C., Knoll, G., Isakov, V., & Modai, I. (2005). Schizophrenia patients with a history of severe violence differ from nonviolent schizophrenia patients in perception of emotions but not cognitive function. *The Journal of Clinical Psychiatry, 66*, 300–308.
Silver, H., & Shlomo, N. (2001). Perception of facial emotions in chronic schizophrenia does not correlate with negative symptoms but correlates with cognitive and motor dysfunction. *Schizophrenia Research, 52*, 265–273.
Simoncelli, E. P., & Olshausen, B. A. (2001). Natural image statistics and neural representation. *Annual Review of Neuroscience, 24*, 1193–1216.
Sini, C. (2014). *Il profondo e l'espressione. Filosofia, psichiatria e psicoanalisi*. IPOC.
Skottun, B. C., & Skoyles, J. R. (2009). Stereopsis and magnocellular sensitivity in schizophrenia. *The World Journal of Biological Psychiatry, 10*, 697–701.
Slaghuis, W. L. (1998). Contrast sensitivity for stationary and drifting spatial frequency gratings in positive- and negative-symptom schizophrenia. *Journal of Abnormal Psychology, 107*, 49–62.
Soames, S. (2012). *Philosophy of language*. Princeton University Press.
Sperber, D., & Wilson, D. (1986). *Relevance: Communication and cognition*. Blackwell.
Stanghellini, G. (2006). *Psicopatologia del senso commune*. Raffaello Cortina Editore.
Stanghellini, G., Ballerini, M., Presenza, S., Mancini, M., Raballo, A., Blasi, S., & Cutting, J. (2016). Psychopathology of lived time: Abnormal time experience in persons with schizophrenia. *Schizophrenia Bulletin, 42*, 46.
Stanley, J. (2007). *Language in context: Selected essays*. Oxford University Press.
Stehen, G. (2004). Can discourse proprieties of metaphor affect metaphor recognition? *Journal of Pragmatics, 36*(7), 1295–1313.
Strawson, P. (1992). *Analyse und metaphysik*. DTV.
Streit, M., Wolwer, W., & Gaebel, W. (1997). Facial-affect recognition and visual scanning behaviour in the course of schizophrenia. *Schizophrenia Research, 24*, 311–317.
Strobl, R., & Resch, F. (1988). Der schizophrene Konkretismus. *Nervenarzt, 59*, 99–102.
Svevo, I. (1923). *La coscienza di Zeno*. Feltrinelli.
Tarski, A., & Corcoran, J. (1923). *Logic, semantics, metamathematics: Papers from 1923 to 1938*. Hackett Publishing Co..
Tartter, V., Gomes, H., & Dubrowsky, B. (2002). Novel metaphors appear anomalous at least momentarily: Evidence from N400. *Brain and Language, 80*(3), 488–509.
Tavano, A. (2008). Specific linguistic and pragmatic deficits in Italian patients with schizophrenia. *Schizophrenia Research, 102*, 59.
Taylor, R. P., Spehar, B., Van Donkelaar, P., & Hagerhall, C. M. (2011). Perceptual and physiological responses to Jackson Pollock's fractals. *Frontiers in Human Neuroscience, 5*, 60.
Thakkar, K. N., & Park, S. (2010). Empathy, schizotypy, and visuospatial transformation. *Cognitive Neuropsychiatry, 15*, 477–500.

Thoma, P., Bauser, D. S., Christine, N., Brüne, M., Juckel, G., & Suchan, B. (2013). Do you see what I feel? – Electrophysiological correlates of emotional face and body perception in schizophrenia. *Clinical Neurophysiology, 125*, 1152–1163.

Thoma, P., & Daum, I. (2006). Neurocognitive mechanisms of figurative language processing – Evidence from clinical dysfunctions. *Neuroscience & Biobehavioral Reviews, 30*, 1182–1205.

Thomas, P., King, K., & Fraser, W. I. (1987). Positive and negative symptoms of schizophrenia and linguistic performance. *Acta Psychiatrica Scandinavica, 76*, 144–151.

Thomas, P., King, K., Fraser, W. I., & Kendell, R. E. (1990). Linguistic performance in schizophrenia: A comparison of acute and chronic patients. *British Journal of Psychiatry, 156*, 204–210.

Travaglini, G. (2009). *Vedere il simile. La metafora, l'anima e le cose in Aristotele*. ETS.

Van Berkum, J. J. A., Hagoort, P., & Brown, C. M. (1999). Semantinc integration in sentences and discourse: Evidence from the N400. *Journal of Cognitive Neuroscience, II*(6), 657–671.

Van Kleeck, M. H. (1989). Hemispheric differences in global versus local processing of hierarchical visual stimuli by normal subjects. *Neuropsychologia, 27*, 1165–1178.

Vaskinn, A., Sundet, K., Østefjells, T., Nymo, K., Melle, I., & Ueland, T. (2016). Reading emotions from body movement: A generalized impairment in schizophrenia. *Frontiers in Psychology, 6*, 1–7.

Vico, G. (1744). *La scienza nuova*. Rizzoli.

Viher, P. V., Stegmayer, K., Kubicki, M., Karmacharya, S., Lyall, A. E., Federspiel, A., Vanbellingen, T., Bohlhalter, S., Wiest, R., Strik, W., & Walther, S. (2017). The cortical signature of impaired gesturing: Findings from schizophrenia. *NeuroImage Clinical, 17*, 213–221.

Vogeley, K., May, M., Ritzl, A., Falkai, P., Zilles, K., & Fink, G. R. (2004). Neural correlates of first-person perspective as one constituent of human self-consciousness. *Journal of Cognitive Neuroscience, 16*, 817–827.

Walker-Smith, G. J., Gale, A. G., & Findlay, J. M. (1977). Eye movement strategies involved in face perception. *Perception, 6*, 313–326.

Warburg, A. (1929). *Atlas mnemosyne*. Ediciones Akal Sa.

Watanabe, S., Kakigi, R., Koyama, S., & Kirino, E. (1999). Human face perception traced by magneto- and electro-encephalography. *Cognitive Brain Research, 8*, 125–142.

Weber, B., Schwarz, U., Kneifel, S., Treyer, V., & Buck, A. (2000). Hierarchical visual processing is dependent on the oculomotor system. *NeuroReport, 11*, 241–247.

Weber, C. S. (2008). *Nasen riechen Tulpen. Kunst von besonderen Menschen im Kontext der Sammlung Würth* (p. 45). Museum Würth und Swiridoff.

Wellman, H., Cross, D., & Watson, J. (2001). Meta-analysis of theory-of-mind development: The truth about false belief. *Child Development, 72*(3), 655–684.

Weniger, G., & Irle, E. (2008). Allocentric memory impaired and egocentric memory intact as assessed by virtual reality in recent-onset schizophrenia. *Schizophrenia Research, 101*, 206.

Werner, H. (1953). *Einführung in die Entwicklungspsychologie*. Barth.

Whittaker, J. F., Deakin, J. F., & Tomenson, B. (2001). Face processing in schizophrenia: Defining the deficit. *Psychological Medicine, 31*, 499–507.

Williams, L. M., Loughland, C. M., Gordon, E., & Davidson, D. (1999). Visual scanpaths in schizophrenia: Is there a deficit in face recognition? *Schizophrenia Research, 40*, 189–199.

Williams, L. M., Loughland, C. M., Green, M. J., Harris, A. W. F., & Gordon, E. (2003). Emotion perception in schizophrenia: An eye movement study comparing the effectiveness of risperidone vs. haloperidol. *Psychiatry Research, 120*, 13–27.

Wilson, D., & Sperber, D. (2012). *Meaning and relevance*. Cambridge University Press.

Wimmer, H., & Perner, J. (1983). Beliefs about beliefs: Representation and contrasting function of wrong beliefs on young children's understanding of deception. *Cognition, 13*(I), 103–128.

Wittgenstein, L. (1921). *Tractatus logico-philosophicus: Logisch-philosophische Abhandlung*. Suhrkamp.

Wittgenstein, L. (1953). *Philosophische Untersuchungen*. Suhrkamp.

Yarbus, A. L. (1967). *Eye movement and vision*. Plenum Press.

Zhang H, Ekstrom A. (2013). Human neural systems underlying rigid and flexible forms of allocentric spatial representation. *Hum Brain Mapp. 34*(5):1070–1087. https://doi.org/10.1002/hbm.21494. Epub 2012 Jan 16. PMID: 22786703; PMCID: PMC6870227.

MIX
Papier aus verantwortungsvollen Quellen
Paper from responsible sources
FSC® C105338

If you have any concerns about our products,
you can contact us on
ProductSafety@springernature.com

In case Publisher is established outside the EU,
the EU authorized representative is:
Springer Nature Customer Service Center GmbH
Europaplatz 3, 69115 Heidelberg, Germany

Printed by Libri Plureos GmbH
in Hamburg, Germany